Joe Barrett is a uniquely spiritual yet down-to-earth fitness devotee who has encapsulated his lifetime of experiences in the realms of bodybuilding, exercise, and nutrition within this enjoyable and informative book. I've worked out in the same gym as Joe for the better part of two decades, and I'm excited that he's decided to share his valuable insights with the rest of the world.

John Phelan, Ph.D.
Professor of Anatomy, University of Texas

This is one of the most important messages of the Bible. Jesus said in John 10:10 "I have come that you might have life and that more abundantly." Life means being healthy.

Bishop Richmond Goodwin, D.D.
Presiding Bishop of the Apostolic Church of Deliverance

This information is a God send. Joseph has definitely addressed a major issue concerning our health. We have to make this a part of our daily routine by applying the principles in this book. This is a process and a lifestyle.

Terrence G. LeGall, CEO / Founder
New Century Investor

Thank you for spreading the word of the complete concept of a healthy mind, body, and spirit.

John Kemper, Founder
Diamond Gym
1981 IFBB World Games Hwy Champ, 1983 NPC Jr.
USA Hwy Champ, 1987 NPC Master's Nat'l Champ

LIVING A

God-Glorifying Life

THROUGH

Good Health

LIVING A
God-Glorifying Life
THROUGH
Good Health

JOSEPH ELIJAH BARRETT

TATE PUBLISHING *& Enterprises*

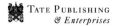
TATE PUBLISHING
& Enterprises

Tate Publishing is committed to excellence in the publishing industry. Our staff of highly trained professionals, including editors, graphic designers, and marketing personnel, work together to produce the very finest books available. The company reflects the philosophy established by the founders, based on Psalms 68:11,

"THE LORD GAVE THE WORD AND GREAT WAS THE COMPANY OF THOSE WHO PUBLISHED IT."

If you would like further information, please contact us:
1.888.361.9473 | www.tatepublishing.com
TATE PUBLISHING & Enterprises, LLC | 127 E. Trade Center Terrace
Mustang, Oklahoma 73064 USA

Published in the United States of America

ISBN: 1-5988690-8-6

07.01.17

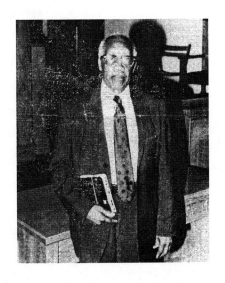

In memory of Elder Joseph Elias Barrett (1898—1987)

Acknowledgements

My father, the late Elder Joseph Elias Barrett, instilled in my subconscious mind a concern for a healthy body as well as a love for God's Word. The foundation that he laid is the basis for this book.

I would also like to recognize and thank my parents collectively. My father, together with my mother, Mrs. Gladys McCloud, provided me with a God-fearing home filled with love. This family background permeates much of this book. I have included many cherished memories based on our family life together in a few of the chapters.

I wish to thank Kenny Morant for suggesting and then encouraging me to write a nutrition and exercise book. Kenny is a bodybuilder who works out at Diamond Gym in Maplewood, NJ.

Table of Contents

Preface

My first step in this book project after having decided to write it was coming up with a suitable title. I knew the subject I would write about. I just had to come up with a descriptive title to reflect it.

The first title I conceived was *Living a God-Glorifying Life in Good Health*. The only difference between this title and the one I finally decided on is one word. I decided on using the word *through* instead of *in*. I saw that there is a difference, however subtle, between the two words. But I believe this difference conveys a powerful truth.

Living a God-Glorifying Life in Good Health implies that it is also possible to lead a God-glorifying life in *bad* health. The premise of this book is that it is not. However, the title *Living a God-Glorifying Life through Good Health* conveys the message that conscious regard for bodily maintenance in and of itself glorifies the Creator. As a matter of fact, conscious regard through nutrition and exercise for the body given us by God is the *only* way that our lives can be God glorifying.

I pray that you the reader will benefit from the contents of these pages so that you may experience the fullness of joy God has for you *in this world*.

Introduction

I think that most Christians are aware that trials and tribulations do not cease once they become born again. As a matter of fact, they seem to increase. Jesus says that no servant is greater than his master (John 13:16). Jesus suffered when He walked the earth and so must we. However, I don't think that those same Christians are as aware of the total freedom and benefits that we have in Christ along with the trials.

Freedom in Christ does not mean that we are free to do as we please with our bodies, or that we are free from trials. We must first realize that our physical bodies do not belong to us. We don't own them. We had nothing whatsoever to do with our existence. We didn't make ourselves, and we didn't cause our birth. God is the reason that we exist. At the same time He has given us the responsibility of maintaining our bodies. When we do that we are guaranteed a quality, happy, and spirit-filled life.

It is against the law to physically abuse children, or for a husband to abuse his wife or for a wife to abuse her husband. God doesn't look kindly on such behavior either. But did you know that there is such a thing as self-abuse? This is the type of abuse that goes unnoticed because it is so common. We all at one time or another have engaged in self-abuse. We just didn't know it.

Self-abuse is not against the law of man, but it is against the law of God!

What constitutes self-abuse? When a person neglects his body (doesn't exercise) such that it becomes susceptible to debilitating illnesses, and feeds it nutrient deficient food (fast and processed food, soda) and poisonous substances (prescription and nonprescription drugs), I define it as self-abuse. Almost everyone is ignorant of this type of abuse. I know I was ignorant of it for most of my life. But now I have no excuse. Now I am aware. And you will become aware after reading this book.

Self-abuse causes damage to God's property. Yes, you, including your body, are God's property. Since we are not our own, we don't have the right to abuse another's property. Actually self-abuse is literally vandalism—the destruction of private property. In this case, the private property being destroyed is the body. And the owner of this property is God.

"Meats for the belly, and the belly for meats: but God shall destroy both it and them. Now the body is not for fornication, *but for the Lord, and the Lord for the body*" (I Corinthians 6:13). Although Paul is addressing fornication, note the italicized phrase, *but for the Lord*. Verse 20 says that we were bought with a price, and that we are to glorify God *in our bodies*. This includes the physical aspect as well as the spiritual.

"Beloved, I wish above all things that thou mayest prosper and be in health, even as thy soul prospereth" (III John 2). "Health" comes from the Greek word *hugiaino*.[1] It signifies to be *sound* or *whole*. "Prosper" is translated from the Greek word *euodoo*.[2] The prefix *eu* means "well." A God of love, like any loving parent, wants the very best for His children.

If the only thing the world saw by watching Christians was poverty, persecution, turmoil, an inability to pay bills, walking around in tattered clothing, and living in shacks, they would think twice about Christianity. Likewise if the world saw the majority of Christians in poor health, constantly complaining about their aches and pains, in and out of the hospital, dependent on multiple prescriptions, they would also think twice about Christianity. I know I would.

Note the above passage of Scripture (III John 2). Seeing that Christians are rich in the spirit, John under the inspiration of the Holy Spirit desires for us to also be blessed with *material* prosperity *and* good health. To miss either one is to miss the abundant life in Christ. God is not glorified by that. Read the words of Jesus Himself. "The thief cometh not, but for to steal, and to kill, and to destroy: I am come that they might have life, and that they might have it *more abundantly*" (John 10:10).

According to the laws of America, ignorance is no excuse. But if Christians are not taught the abundant life in Christ, they *can* plead ignorance. But they will pay the price. They will fail to reap the full benefits of a committed Christian life. The purpose of this book is to point out how Christians can and should live in complete health. (There are many fine books that share the material and financial aspect of the abundant life, and we therefore will not go into it here). Once it is understood what God demands *of* you, and you implement the steps discussed, you will begin to reap the benefits God has *for* you.

The foundation on which the care of the body is based is first established. The body is a gift from God and we have been entrusted with its stewardship (management). Therefore it is incumbent upon us to take care of the body. Its maintenance is a two-fold process. It consists of physical exercise *and* nutrition. They must both go hand-in-hand. The need is greater now than it was even a few short years ago.

I know that for some people "exercise" is a four-letter word. I know you are not one of them. For others, excuses are plentiful when reminded of it. Having exercised consistently for about thirty years (I started by running, and then lifting weights in 1978), I've heard many an excuse and some have been doozies. "I don't have the time," "My (husband, wife, friend) stopped going with me," "I'm too tired," "The weather's too bad outside" (when I suggest the mall, the excuse becomes "I'll stop to shop"), and on and on and on. Recognize yourself? Don't feel bad. I've been there.

But when we begin to realize the care that God used in preparing the physical universe for the body, and then how carefully

He made the body from the soil, we get a whole new mind set. We *take* the time to exercise just as we *take* the time to breathe. (I hope that point is not lost on anyone.) One of the ways to please God is by taking care of the body through exercise and good nutrition. This is just as important as fasting and praying and all the other spiritual gifts we offer up to God.

I purchased a brand new Ford Explorer in 1999. Included with the new SUV was an owner's manual. This manual contains everything the owner should know and be aware of concerning his vehicle. It not only describes every feature, but, if appropriate, how to set or change it, and how to operate it. The manual also specifies which grade of gasoline to use, whether regular, middle, or premium.

The owner's manual also comes with a complete maintenance schedule. This schedule tells you what should be done at certain, predetermined vehicle miles. When it is followed, the new SUV, or whatever type of vehicle it is, should give years of trouble free service.

Where did the owner's manual come from? In my case it came from the Ford Motor company, the creator of the Explorer. As the maker of the Explorer, Ford is thoroughly familiar with it. They designed it to operate optimally on a certain grade of gasoline, and to be driven in a certain way and under certain circumstances. If I have any questions about my Explorer, I wouldn't seek answers from my local auto body shop, or a Chevy dealer for that matter. I would call my local Ford dealer.

Who but God is qualified to know everything there is to know about a human being—spirit, soul, and body? Concerning the body, God knows what will keep it functioning and in perfect health. As with a new car, our bodies have a maintenance schedule. Follow it and we will be rewarded with good health. Deviate from it, and the body at some point in time will break down.

The maintenance schedule for the body is one that everyone follows in varying degrees. Most people, though, are not thorough enough and skip certain steps while others use the wrong ingredients. If our cars are maintained in the same slipshod manner in which we maintain our bodies, I can almost guarantee big time trouble down the road.

Maintenance consists of two phases: exercise *and* nutrition. We all eat on a daily basis. We just don't all eat the correct number of times and use the right food in the proper amount. And exercise has become little to none at all. Muscles and the cardiovascular system, like a car's engine, have to be kept in tune (as with the memory, you either *use it or lose it*).

There are certain universal spiritual principles operating in this world. These spiritual principles will benefit the sinner as well as the saint. In Matthew 5:45 Jesus says, "That ye may be the children of your Father which is in heaven: for he maketh his sun to rise on the evil and on the good, and sendeth rain on the just and on the unjust." A person who gives unselfishly to those who are less fortunate will be wealthy—they will prosper. Solomon says as much in the following quote from the book of Ecclesiastes: "Cast thy bread upon the waters: for thou shalt find it after many days" (11:1).

Likewise, good health will benefit anyone who follows God's maintenance schedule for the human body. Unfortunately it seems as though many people, Christians included, have put physical health on the back burner. For others it is an afterthought. Although a healthy body will not benefit a Christian beyond this life, it will glorify God in this world as it is *His dwelling place*. "What? Know ye not that your body is the temple of the Holy Ghost which is in you, which ye have of God, and ye are not your own?" (I Corinthians 6:19).

As children of the King, God wants the best for us. He desires for us to prosper and flourish in this life financially, physically, and mentally, as much as we are prospering in our spirit man. Third John 2 bears repeating. "Beloved, I wish above all things that thou mayest prosper and be in health, even as thy soul prospereth."

God receives no glory from a body that is constantly getting sick, being hospitalized, and pumped full of synthetic man-made chemicals (commonly known as prescription drugs) because it was fed incorrectly, and not given regular tune-ups (exercise). Our being miserable, in pain, and forced to spend our meager, hard-earned money for over-priced medication is not the type of suffering that glorifies God.

The abuse and/or neglect of the body, which God in His infinite wisdom so carefully crafted, saddens our Heavenly Father. The children of the King are to reflect the King. Our God is *not* poor and sick, but rich and flawless. The royal family of England does not go about as paupers and looking like ragamuffins. They are royalty and look and act like royalty. Likewise we are royalty. Our God is King of kings and Lord of lords. "But ye are a chosen generation, a royal priesthood, an holy nation, a peculiar people; that ye should shew forth the praises of him who hath called you out of darkness into his marvellous light" (I Peter 2:9).

Let me ask you a question. What good is it for a Christian to have material and financial wealth and a weak and sick body? In all probability this body also needs multiple prescriptions for several, and I might add preventable, health issues. The Christian living the full abundant life in Christ should be materially wealthy and having no health issues at all. None! And age does not enter into the equation at all. The body at 80, 90, and even 100 years old should be as healthy and fit as a body in its 20s, 30s, or 40s. I know—you're shaking your head in stark disbelief and astonishment. You think that I am a looney. Follow the guidelines in this book and I can assure you that this can be you. You want a living example? Look at Jack LaLanne!

Dr. Don Colbert, a Christian with a family medical practice in Orlando, Florida, reevaluated his lifestyle after developing chronic fatigue syndrome and psoriasis. He started to investigate the connection between physical, spiritual, and mental health. Dr. Colbert eliminated all processed foods from his diet, and started an exercise program. His health improved dramatically.

Dr. Colbert did not stop at diet and exercise. He stopped prescribing so many prescription drugs and instead suggested lifestyle and diet changes to his patients. Dr. Colbert now embraces alternative medicine. Says Dr. Colbert, ". . . Jesus, his apostles and others of their time got plenty of exercise in the course of their normal lives, equivalent to walking three to ten miles daily. . . "[3]
In thinking back over my life, I realize that I ate a lot of junk.

Refined sugar, cakes, cookies, candies, and white rice and breads galore were my daily diet. I was also a soda drinker early on. I gave up soda decades ago. My consumption of other sweets has gone down considerably, too. I can truthfully say that I have never been on either prescription or nonprescription drugs. This is one of the contributing factors to the state of my health today. *I don't get sick!* Many of the health issues today stem from a steady diet of synthetic prescription and nonprescription drugs, processed foods, and no exercise. I can guarantee you that by eliminating refined sugar, processed and junk foods, and prescription and nonprescription medication from your diet, and implementing an exercise program and eating whole, organic food, the body will begin to heal itself.

Prescription drugs and processed foods are why so many people suffer from asthma, high blood pressure, migraine headaches, osteoporosis, digestive problems, various forms of cancer, heart disease, and so on and so forth. Synthetic and foreign chemicals are being shoved into God's all natural body. The body's cells are being subjected to unnatural substances, and confusion arises. Remember this one point if you don't remember anything else. Man's prescription and nonprescription drugs cannot cure anything. All they do is to treat the symptom by suppressing it while the cause of that symptom goes undiagnosed. This way Big Pharma can keep you on their medications for life. Only God's all natural and organic foods can allow the body to heal itself. By eliminating the cause, you eliminate the symptom. It's as simple as that.

A recent Time Magazine article reported on a study conducted by the Harvard School of Public Health. The study concerned the number of cancer cases for which obesity was the cause. The total number of cases reported was 100,000 per year. I suspect that this is a conservative number. Here's the breakdown by cancer type:

Breast cancer: 11%
Colon cancer: 14%
Endometrial cancer: 49%

Esophageal cancer: 39%
Kidney cancer: 31%
Non-Hodgkin's lymphoma: 20%
Pancreatic cancer: 14%

The *Journal of the American Medical Association* (JAMA) recently ran an article concerning the results of its study of the comparative health of white middle-aged Americans versus their contemporaries in England. These results should provide a wake-up call to all Americans. Regardless of education and income level, white middle-aged Americans have higher rates of diabetes, heart disease, strokes, lung disease, and cancer than their British counterparts. This is true despite the fact that America spends about twice as much money on health care as do the English! Specifically, this shocking study showed that diabetes was twice as high in America and cancer was almost twice as high as compared with the rate found among the English. Dr. Joseph Mercola remarks, "For one thing, 90% of the money Americans spend on food goes towards processed foods. . . How can you possibly be healthy with that much processed food in your diet?"[4]

This book is over thirty years in the making. About thirty years ago while watching TV I saw a Dannon yogurt commercial. This commercial was touting the longevity enhancing ingredients of Dannon yogurt by looking at the Russian people of Soviet Georgia. The name of the commercial, which aired from 1975 to 1978, was *Old People In Russia.* This commercial claimed that the extraordinary life spans of these people were due to the yogurt in their diet.

A people group called Hunzas who have been studied by Western medical doctors does exist. These people who live high in the mountains of northern Pakistan are among the longest living people groups in the entire world. They routinely live to b e 100 to 120 years old, and beyond.

I was so overwhelmed and inspired by the Hunza people that I decided to start an exercise program. I later added Dannon yogurt to my diet, although not because of the claims made by Dannon. I began jogging. I started in the early to mid 70s and kept increasing my distance until I reached the ten mile point. Before I started jogging I played basketball after school on a somewhat regular basis.

In 1978 I started lifting weights (bodybuilding). I stopped running shortly afterwards because engaging in both activities was too much. My goal through bodybuilding was to increase my size and weight. I had a very fast metabolism and was very thin for my height (5' 10"). I accomplished both goals. Starting at a body weight of about 150 pounds, I reached a top weight of 212 pounds.

During my early bodybuilding days I entered several physique competitions. This is where I learned a lot about dieting. I would successfully diet down to a competitive weight of about 175 pounds. After the show, I would intentionally gain 20 to 25 pounds. The weight gain though was mostly muscle since I did lift weights 4 to 6 days a week.

Bodybuilding also taught me a lot about nutrition. I began reading books and magazines about different exercises, and the importance of supplementation and good nutrition. I avoided all steroids and other synthetic performance enhancing drugs. I started and remained all natural. I have read about and have personally known bodybuilders who have died directly or indirectly through synthetic drug use.

This book contains over thirty years of my personal experience, knowledge, and observations. Coupled with my study of the Bible and Christian walk of well over twenty years, it can change your life. The only variable is you. Are you ready to acknowledge the fact that you shouldn't be feeling as bad as you do most of the time? Are you ready to acknowledge the fact that you shouldn't have to take prescription and nonprescription drugs? Are you ready to acknowledge the fact that you shouldn't be out of breath after walking up only one flight of stairs? Are you ready to acknowledge the fact that you are going to the hospital much too often? Are you tired of feeling "pooped" and sluggish all day? Are you tired of feeling stressed out? Are you sick and tired of being sick and tired? If the answer to all of these questions is yes, and you apply exercise and good nutrition to your life, then prepare to feel like you've never felt before, and be as healthy as a Hunza. And yes, as healthy as I am.

This book is not a "how-to" book. You will not find detailed exercise programs in it. Neither is it a book of suggested meal plans. However, I do make a few suggestions for exercise routines. But in general, exercise and meal specifics are beyond the scope of this book. My primary concern is to point out from a biblical vantage point that we are to be as aware of our physical life as we are of our spiritual life.

As a baby boomer growing up in America I have seen a lot of technological change. I realize that change is inevitable. As a matter of fact, the only thing in this society that won't change is the fact that things will change. Man will continue to progress and improve the way we do things. He will also invent new machines and devices to save time and labor.

However, there is a downside to change or progress. It is unfortunate that this downside is not always apparent when a new process or gadget is implemented. We are reaping these multiplied downsides today in devastating ways. The new technology of yesteryear is compromising our health and sending us to early graves today.

Growing up in the 50s and 60s we, like today's youth, ate hot dogs and hamburgers and drank sodas and shoved tons of cakes, cookies and ice cream down our throats. Despite all of this junk food we remained "slim and trim" and didn't have the medical crisis so common today. What's changed? That question can be answered in one word—technology! Trans fat, which has turned out to be the worst fat ever, didn't appear in the commercial market until the early to mid 80s. They replaced what was thought to be responsible for clogged arteries and high cholesterol—saturated fats. The first microwave oven for home use was manufactured by Amana, a subsidiary of Raytheon, in 1967. HFCS (High Fructose Corn Syrup) was introduced as a sweetener in the 1970s. Passive devices such as cell phones and video games and computers (through which we access the internet) are relatively latecomers (mid to late 80s and later).

Television and radio were the only forms of electronic entertainment back in the days of us baby boomers. Contrast that with today. After watching several hours of television, today's youth have their video games, cell phones, and computers to provide entertainment and diversion. They don't have the time or the inclination to play or exercise. More soda is being consumed today than ever before. And because of all the sweeteners and HFCS, today's soda is not only addictive but health threatening as well.

There has also been an explosion of fast food franchises in addition to new franchises sprouting up. Along with fast food restaurants there has been a rabbit like growth of drug stores. The food industry has produced hundreds of processed foods to appeal to consumer taste buds and reduce time in the kitchen. The following chapters will provide details on how these innovations negatively impact your life.

The following chapters will also describe to you in detail how you can change your mind set to what it should be. Your spirit and soul have been liberated. Now it is time to whip the third part of man, the body, into a God-glorifying vessel. "And the very God of peace sanctify you wholly; and I pray God your whole spirit and soul and *body* be preserved blameless unto the coming of our Lord Jesus Christ" (I Thessalonians 5:23).

CHAPTER 1

The Body in the Beginning

MAN'S BODY

After God finished creating everything, He made the following assessment, "And God saw everything that he had made, and, behold, it was very good. And the evening and the morning were the sixth day" (Genesis 1:31). There was no flaw or imperfection in anything that God had made, and that includes man.

In five verses prior to Genesis 1:31 we see the statement "and God saw that it was good" written (Genesis 1:10, 12, 18, 21, 25). This means that not only was each act of creation perfect, and complete within the range God ordained for it, but that it gave God *pleasure*—He was thoroughly satisfied. I compare this feeling to the feeling I get when I write, compose, and design a magazine or book. It's a deep sense of gratification that can only come from something that you are personally responsible for. You sit back and enjoy it, reflecting on the work and creativity that went into it. This feeling is hard to explain—it has to be experienced to be understood.

"And the Lord God formed man of the dust of the ground, and breathed into his nostrils the breath of life; and man became a living soul" (Genesis 2:7). Genesis 2:7 shows that God did something unique to man that He didn't do even to angels. After He had formed man from the earth's clay, He actually *imparted* Himself into man by breathing into him. By that single act, man became intimately associated with God. So you see not one part of the three-fold being of man can be lightly esteemed or neglected, whether it is spirit, soul, *or body*.

God derived extreme joy and pleasure from each act of creation. The Supreme Being who is the Ultimate Reality and the all-powerful, all knowing, everywhere present One who has no beginning was gratified with not only the heavens and the earth, but especially with man himself. Man is the only living creature, with the possible exception of angels, whom God made to enjoy eternal fellowship with.

The fact that at five different times God stopped and looked at what he had just created and put His "seal of approval" on it suggests extreme love and devotion. Neither creation nor man was a rush job. To knowingly abuse our bodies, which are a source of pride for God, and which demonstrate His love, is unthinkable. It is our duty to protect our environment *and* our bodies!

Evidence strongly suggests that Adam and early man, as well as animals and plant life, were huge—veritable giants. Fossil remains indicate that animals besides dinosaurs grew to enormous sizes. Ancient plants and insects were also larger than those that thrive today.

Genesis 2:7 describes how God molded man from the dust of the earth. This was not the earth of today ravaged with pollution and depleted of vital nutrients. The earth then was perfect. That means that Adam's body was a perfect physical body. It was healthy, and germ and toxin free. "I will praise thee; for I am fearfully and wonderfully made: marvelous are thy works; and that my soul knoweth right well" (Psalms 139:14).

Not only would Adam's physical size dwarf that of modern man, but his body far exceeded ours in health and vitality, both internally and externally. His huge muscles and low body fat levels would make today's most elite athlete look anemic in comparison.

Adam and Eve's superior health, complexion, and immune system would shock today's medical profession. Medical textbooks would have to be rewritten. Standard tests would have to be re-evaluated. What is considered normal and healthy today would be far surpassed if physicians could travel back in time and give Adam and Eve a physical. As a matter of fact, the results of their complete physical examination would have to become the new standard of normality for man today.

God designed our bodies to be sustained by natural food and water. "And out of the ground made the Lord God to grow every tree that is pleasant to the sight, and *good for food. . .* " (Genesis 2:9a). He did not make the body to be nourished by processed and manufactured food. God provided natural herbs, plant and marine life, as well as various minerals, to assist the body in repairing and healing itself, and to provide fuel. God did foresee that man's exploding technology would cause harmful and often deadly physical side effects, but His original creation is the only food that the body can assimilate without any long-term damage.

One thing many people fail to realize is that they don't own their bodies. It is owned by the Creator. Adam and his posterity were given the mandate to manage the earth. "And God blessed them, and God said unto them, Be fruitful, and multiply, and replenish [*fill, populate*] the earth, and subdue it: and have dominion over the fish of the sea, and over the fowl of the air, and over every living thing that moveth upon the earth" (Genesis 1:28). Man also has the responsibility to manage his body. We didn't make our bodies and therefore we don't have the luxury or the right of doing anything that we please to them. *God desires for you to prosper and be in health!*

MAN'S FOOD

Originally man's food was totally natural and organic. "And God said, Behold, I have given you every *herb bearing seed*, which is upon the face of all the earth, and *every tree, in the which is the fruit of a tree yielding seed*; to you it shall be for meat [food]" (Genesis 1:29).

Before Adam's sin, man's diet consisted only of "every herb bearing seed" (grains, seeds, nuts, and legumes) and "every tree, in which is the fruit of a tree yielding fruit" (apples, pears, etc). Grains are wheat, corn, rye, barley, rice, etc. Seeds comprise sunflower, sesame, flax, etc. Legumes are soybeans, peas, beans, etc. There are various types of nuts: almonds, pecans, walnuts and many others. Notice that the green herb *was not* a part of man's diet before sin.

Genesis 3:18 records the first item God added to man's post-sin diet, the green herb. "Thorns also and thistles shall it bring forth to thee; and thou shalt *eat the herb of the field*." In the beginning only animals ate these green herbs or vegetables. The second item that God included in man's diet was meat. "Every moving thing that liveth shall be meat for you; even as the green herb have I given you all things" (Genesis 9:3).

The plants, fruits, and veggies back in those days were physically perfect. As with man and animals, they were much larger than their modern counterparts. Plant life then did not grow in vitamin- and mineral-depleted soil. They also didn't have to be certified organic by government agencies because God Himself saw that everything was *very good*.

Foods were not bleached white in order to appeal to the eye. There also were no programs researching ways to prolong shelf life, or to find chemical additives in order to get people addicted to processed food (which studies have shown create medical problems). The plants and fruits of those early days were replete with minerals and vitamins.

Because the plants and fruit were complete and not tampered with, there was no need for early man to supplement his diet. Supplementation is needed today. Doctors, insurance companies, and hospitals were not needed either. Man's health didn't fail him because pharmaceutical companies producing toxic, synthetic drugs did not exist. There was no need for synthetic drugs because man was satisfied with what God had provided. He didn't see a need to seek alternatives, or ways to improve it. Remember, no one knows more about a creation than its Creator. God made man and everything else. No one, whether doctor, pharmaceutical company, or scientist, knows more about the human body, or its health, than God. *God desires for you to prosper and be in health!*

ANIMAL'S FOOD

God created land animals and insects on day 6, the same day that man was made (Genesis 1:24–31). Fish and birds were created on day 5 (Genesis 1:20–22). The food for all land animals, including the insects, and for all birds is the green herb. "And to every beast of the earth, and to every fowl of the air, and to every thing that creepeth upon the earth, wherein there is life, I have given *every green herb* for meat: and it was so" (Genesis 1:30).

The green herbs that God gave to birds, land animals, and insects are vegetables. They include leafy vegetables such as beet greens, Brussels sprouts, and cabbage. Another type of green herb is classified as "flower." This includes the globe artichoke, broccoli, and cauliflower. The third type of green herb is known as "root." This type includes carrots, beets, and turnips.

The eating habits and patterns of land animals, birds, and insects today are totally different from those before man sinned. Today we know that many animals are carnivorous (meat-eaters). Mosquitoes include blood in their diet.

WATER

The water supply in God's original creation was nontoxic and pollution free. It was nothing like our modern "tap" water. The waters on the earth of Adam's day and even that of the Hebrew patriarchs was natural and pure. There were no pollutants and industrial waste to contaminate it. Remember, God saw that it was good.

When I was growing up in the 50s and early 60s, water was free. And our only source was the water company. Unlike today, water wasn't sold in stores just as air wasn't sold at gas stations. Although fluoride and chlorine were already being mixed into the water supply by the nation's water companies, the potential dangers were not then known.

Chemicals, notably fluoride and chlorine, have been added to drinking water to combat impurities. But the chemicals fluoride and chlorine are deadly poisons themselves.

"In summary, we hold that fluoridation is an unreasonable risk. That is, the toxicity of fluoride is so great and the purported benefits associated with it are so small—if there are any at all— that requiring every man, woman and child in America to ingest it borders on criminal behavior on the part of governments".[5] Fluoridation of America's water supply began in Grand Rapids, Michigan, in 1945.

Drinking water is also chlorinated. And like fluoride, it is a poison. Studies have found that known carcinogens (cancer causing agents) are in our drinking water because of chlorination. Dr. J.M. Price, MD of Saginaw Hospital says the following, "Chlorine is the greatest crippler and killer of modern times. While it prevented epidemics of one disease, it was creating another. Two decades ago, after the start of chlorinating our drinking water in 1904, the present epidemic of heart trouble, cancer, and senility began"[6]

The *International Journal of Cancer* reported on a group of studies which showed the effect of tap water on men. The results of six control studies involving 2,749 bladder cancer cases and 5,150 cancer free controls revealed that a high consumption of ordinary tap water will slightly increase men's risk of contracting bladder cancer. The risk of bladder cancer increased by 50 percent when men drank more than 2 liters (a little more than ½ gallon) of tap water daily.

Water is imperative for good health. It is used for many internal processes. ". . . Water is vital to digestion and metabolism, acting as a medium for various enzymatic and chemical reactions in the body. It carries nutrients and oxygen to the cells through the blood, regulates body temperature and lubricates our joints. . ."[7]

The human body itself is over 65% water. If the body does not get enough water, excess body fat, poor muscle tone and size, and increased toxicity is the result. Not only is the quantity of water important, but quality also. When the quality of water is compromised, your health also suffers. *God desires for you to prosper and be in health!*

LONGEVITY

Early man lived a lot longer than man does today. Although much of ancient man's longevity could be attributed to a perfect world without sin, man who lived after sin had marred God's creation still lived longer on average than modern man.

Pre-sin man lived for centuries. Adam lived to be 930 years old while his son Seth lived to be 912. The man who had human history's longest life span was Methuselah. He lived to be 969 years old!

After sin and the flood life spans dwindled tremendously. But until very recently, long lives were not spent on prescription drugs and in the care of nursing homes. I am not ridiculing those on prescription drugs or those who are confined to nursing homes. Many are victims of advancing technology and man's greed. Both, however, work against the human body. There will be more on the technological and greed issues later.

When Abraham was 100 years old, he was told by God that he would have a son. "Then Abraham fell upon his face, and laughed, and said in his heart, Shall a child be born unto him that is an hundred years old? And shall Sarah, that is ninety years old, bear?" (Genesis 17:17). Abraham lived to be 175 years old. His son Isaac died at 180.

Moses lived to be 110 years old. Even at that advanced age the Bible says that he had 20/20 vision and he still had the vitality and strength of a much younger person (Deuteronomy 34:7).

These men and women lived long and healthy lives because their food was all natural and organic. They also didn't spend hours living a sedentary life. Their daily routine required them to walk miles, and perform routine activities such as farming and washing, all without the use of labor-saving machines.

Because man lived in an environment free from pollution, artificial food, and chemically treated water, cancer and heart disease were unheard of. His society also didn't have to cope with health threatening obesity, artery clogging fast food, osteoarthritis, or the many other health issues running wild today.

"The days of our years are threescore years and ten; and if by reason of strength they be fourscore years, yet is their strength labour and sorrow; for it is soon cut off, and we fly away" (Psalms 90:10). "Threescore and ten" years is 70 while fourscore is 80. Many people today are living well into their 70s, 80s, and 90s. My father lived to be 87 years old. Although people are living longer today than they did during the last few hundred years, what is the quality of these lives?

First of all, longer lives can be attributed to better medical practices, and better knowledge and nutrition. By better medical practices I don't mean by the introduction of prescription and nonprescription drugs. I refer to new surgical procedures, germ control and sanitary practices.

Better medical knowledge existed thousands of years ago but was forgotten when civilizations forgot God and the Bible. The ancient Israelites had superior medical knowledge because they obeyed the law of God. The books of Numbers, Leviticus, and Deuteronomy contain sanitary practices that God commanded the Israelites to carry out (See Numbers 19, Leviticus 11, 15, and Deuteronomy 23:12–13). They were also given strict guidelines as to quarantining people with infectious diseases (Read Leviticus 13, 14, 22 for the laws of leprosy).

We are living longer on average than people in the 18th and 19th centuries, but are the quality of these lives acceptable? Many people in the United States today are taking multiple prescription and nonprescription drugs. That means they have significant health issues. Some of these are life threatening. But since all prescription and nonprescription drugs are synthetic, and therefore toxic, it is a possibility of the so-called cure being worse then the disease. These drugs may mask the symptom of the medical problem but they don't address the underlying cause of that problem. So while these drugs mask one symptom, they at the same time are responsible for causing other problems down the road.

I don't think there has been any study to correlate longer lives with prescription and nonprescription drug use exclusively. But even if a correlation can be shown, can the practice be condoned because life spans are being increased? No it can't. The longer lives are not *quality* lives. And the key to a God-glorifying life is *quality*, and not *quantity at the expense of quality*. Prescription and nonprescription drugs are poisoning and crippling the body that God so lovingly gave us. It is physical abuse of the worse kind.

Life spans can definitely be increased if the body were not poisoned and neglected. 16th century Spanish explorer Ponce de Leon is credited with searching for the fountain of youth. He didn't have to look any further than the Bible and his own body. Talk about a fountain of youth. Nutrition and physical exercise *is* the fountain of youth.

With proper nutrition and exercise lives would be quality lives. People would not be walking chemical factories! God desires for us to live, and not merely exist and go through the motions of life.

This means that we should have meaningful and productive lives well into our 80s, 90s, and yes, even the 100s! And when we do expire, it would not be with disease riddled bodies, or dementia. Neither would it be tucked away in some nursing home unable to care for ourselves. Again, I am not ridiculing nursing homes or any other health care facility. Unfortunately we need them in America. But wouldn't it be great if we didn't need them? And we wouldn't need them if we could eliminate the cause of their existence. This is possible despite the claims to the contrary by Big Pharma, the food industry, and the so-called health care industry (it could more aptly be called the "sick-care" industry).

I briefly mentioned the Hunzas in the Introduction. The diseases which America thinks are the normal signs of aging are not found in Hunza society. They have no nursing or senior citizen homes. That's because they don't get sick. They don't even catch colds or come down with the flu.

"... Here people lived to be 100, 110, 120, and occasionally as much as 140 years of age. Here lies the real Fountain of Youth—probably the only one in the world. ... Hunza land is truly a Utopia if ever there was one. Just think of this! Here is a land where people do not have our common diseases such as heart ailments, cancer, arthritis, high blood pressure, diabetes, tuberculosis, hay fever, asthma, liver trouble, gall bladder trouble, constipation or many other ailments that plague the rest of the world. . ."[8]

Seems impossible? Does it sound hard to believe? It only seems impossible and hard to believe because all we know in America is sickness, dementia, drugs, and hospitals. We have been brainwashed to believe that this is normal—that this is a normal part of living. I say baloney. And you can throw some salami in there, too. God's Word says we are to *prosper and be in health!*

The Hunza's longevity and absolute health can be attributed to nutrition and hard work from the cradle to the grave. When I was at Elizabethtown Gas Company, I found out that a couple of the retirees died soon after retiring. I remember thinking at the time that they worked hard all their lives and they now faced retirement. They then lived a completely leisurely and sedentary lifestyle. Man was not made to sit and waste away. God made man to work and be productive throughout his entire lifetime.

Hunza water is natural and pure mountain water. They don't add chlorine and fluoride to it like we do. Their food is 100% unprocessed and organic. They don't try to improve the natural food that God has given us. Oh, did I mention that they don't have Burger Kings, White Castles, McDonald's, KFCs or any other fast food restaurants? There is absolutely nothing in their diet that does not originate in nature.

A large part of the Hunza's protein and fat needs are plant in origin. They eat plenty of organic fruits, veggies, and grains, and very little meat. Doesn't this remind you of Genesis 1:29? "And God said, Behold, I have given you every herb bearing seed, which is upon the face of all the earth, and every tree, in the which is the fruit of a tree yielding seed; TO YOU IT SHALL BE FOR MEAT."

No matter how far technology progresses—and what great discoveries scientists and medical doctors make—what God has created and provided for man's body will never be improved by technology.

The other contributing factor to the Hunza's longevity is exercise. They don't need the formalized exercise programs that we in the west need because they don't have the technological advances which remove work (I cover this in detail in the next chapter). Hunza's live high (8,000 ft.) in the Himalayan mountains and they are farmers.

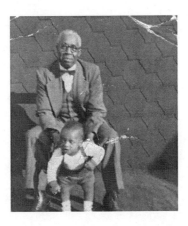

My father Elder Joseph Elias Barrett and yours truly

Hunza men are amazingly strong even into the years where most Americans are frail and intimidated by life. They are said to even father children into their 80s and 90s. Their stamina is also astounding. They walk a lot. Living on mountain slopes, men and women have to walk up and down slopes carrying heavy loads. Here is a quote from an article carried in many major North American newspapers a while back: "...Hunza men over 90 years old reportedly walk the mountain trail of 65 miles from the town of Gilgit with a full pack and immediately start to work in the fields again..."[9]

I don't remember my father as ever being sick, or having to take any type of medication. He never needed any care and certainly never had to be placed in a nursing home. He was born in 1898, and he was 53 years old when I was born. He was 63 years old when the last of his 10 children was born. Other than a foot injury he suffered in a motorcycle accident during World War I, I don't think that he ever had surgery or was ever hospitalized.

What a health record. To be completely honest, I don't think that my father ever went to a doctor's office, or ever had a checkup or physical. I don't mean to suggest that getting a health checkup is a no-no—it's not—it's just that I don't think my father was partial to doctors. And if he wasn't then I inherited it because I'm not particularly partial to doctors either.

I'll always remember my father as disapproving of the overweight and obese people of God he saw at church on Sundays. He wasn't bashful about telling it to them either. Though I'm sure many were offended and annoyed, he was genuinely concerned.

As I reflect upon my father and how he brought us up and the example he set for us, I can see why I am so health oriented. Although this aspect of my life lay dormant in my early years, it has surfaced strongly over the last few years. When I went to Newark College of Engineering in 1970 (it is now known as the New Jersey Institute of Technology), I was influenced to experiment with smoking and drinking. Thank God that I never became physically addicted to either. I did smoke marijuana, too. But as abruptly as I picked it up, I gave it up. My drug use didn't progress to anything else. My health was never impaired because I didn't abuse my body to the point that permanent damage was done. My upbringing was the anchor that stopped the deadly plunge before serious damage was done.

I suspect you may think that I am a fanatic. I guess that I am in a manner of speaking. When it comes to respecting the temple of the Holy Ghost, and my home training, I am as serious as a heart attack. There was a 50s sitcom on television called *Father Knows Best*. When it came to being led by the Spirit of God, my father knew best. And he led by example. *God desires for you to prosper and be in health*!

CHAPTER 2:

Technology and Declining Health

INTRODUCTION

Webster's dictionary defines *technology* as "the science or study of the practical or industrial arts, applied sciences, etc. . . . the system by which a society provides its members with those things needed or desired."

Because of rapidly advancing technology, we can go further faster, produce more food, and see and talk to anyone anywhere in the world in real time. These innovations have been a boon to mankind. But technology has also resulted in a negative trend. We tend to rely on it *too much*!

There is nothing wrong with technology. It is not evil. There is nothing wrong with money either. The Bible says that the *love* of money is the root of all evil (I Timothy 6:10), not the money itself. It is our reaction to technology, like that to money, which can result in harm, or prove harmful.

In this chapter I will list and discuss technological advances that have made our lives easier, but because of "abuse" removed the healthful aspects of the manual labor they replaced. I don't mean abuse in a bad way. This is not a salvation issue. By abuse I mean overuse to the point where all physical benefits have been completely taken away. We have become overly dependent on them.

THE AUTOMOBILE

"...We have always had a very plentiful supply of cheap food," Morgan Downey, head of the American Obesity Association told the BBC. "And we are fascinated with labour-saving devices like the automobile. These are hallmarks of our society and of our problem..."[10]

No one will deny that the automobile is one of the greatest single inventions in all of recorded human history. Travel time has been reduced from weeks and months to days, and sometimes hours or minutes, because of it. Yet the problem is that we have become too dependent on it. We have abused motorized transportation. We will drive our cars to go to the corner store located on the same block on which we live. And what about the malls? People will literally fight for the opportunity to park as close to the entrance as possible—even if they have to park illegally, or in spots designated for the handicapped! No doubt if they could park in the lobby, they would. What a sad commentary on contemporary America!

And what is the trade-off for the misuse of the automobile? We lose the opportunity to walk. Walking is a great form of exercise. It is great for cardiovascular conditioning and weight control (which means weight loss for a great majority of people). We are already a nation of overfed, under exercised people. And now we refuse to engage in an easy and non-stressful form of exercise.

In countries where cars are owned by the wealthy few, or they are only used when necessary, people on average walk much more than we do in America. Americans average less than a mile a day whereas people in other nations average miles. No wonder we are a nation of overweight and obese individuals with bulging waistlines. We are eating more (mostly the wrong kinds of foods) and exercising less, if at all.

A recent editorial in the Washington Post said the following, "... do the math - invest 30 minutes of walking a day and you'll spend 49 days of the next 12 years of your life walking to gain 1.3 healthy years... That's a great payoff, considering that it is also likely the walking will help you keep off fat and improve your mood... Walkers have less incidence of cancer, heart disease, stroke, diabetes and other killer diseases. They live longer and get mental health and spiritual benefits. . . "[11]

Let me give you a page from my life history. I want you to know you that I don't just talk the talk, but that I also walk the walk. I recently had to leave my Ford Explorer at a body shop for repairs to the rear bumper. When I left my truck at the shop, I was asked if I needed a ride home. I said "no." The attendant then asked me if I was sure. I said "yes," I was sure. Now this body shop is about ½ mile from where I live. I could easily have followed the path of least resistance and gotten a ride home. But I declined. Actually I looked forward to the walk. Would you have done the same? Be honest now. If your answer was "no," I am praying that by the time you've finished reading this book, you, too, will look forward to walking more.

Living a God-glorifying life involves spirit, body, and soul. Being dependent on prescription drugs, and held captive by poor eating habits and a refusal to provide daily "maintenance" (exercise) for the temple of the Holy Ghost does not reflect our Savior. It is a trick of the enemy.

Although we are on earth for a very short time while preparing for eternity, God desires His children to live quality lives. We are not to neglect the body He so carefully formed and provided for. Remember, God created man's environment before He placed man in it. When He formed Adam from the 'dust of the earth,' his physical body had everything needed for comfort, pleasure, and sustenance. This illustrates that the body God has given us is not to be tucked away in a corner and forgotten while we pursue more "spiritual" goals.

God has a plan for each and every one of us. That plan can

only be completely fulfilled when we are physically capable of performing it. How could the apostle Paul have fulfilled his mission if he was overweight, and couldn't walk a couple of miles without doubling over from exhaustion and pain? What if his body suffered from high blood pressure, heart disease, type 2 diabetes and other crippling medical problems brought on by lack of exercise and poor eating habits? He probably would have died prematurely before establishing all of the churches we read about in the New Testament! Can you imagine the New Testament part of your Bible missing such books as Romans, Ephesians, or Galatians?

In saying all of this I am not minimizing the importance of the automobile. It is a necessity in today's society. I would be the first to admit it. But at the same time I will not allow it to deprive my body of the exercise I need. Remember the adage 'use it or lose it?' Well it's true. Unused or under utilized muscles will atrophy and grow weak. God desires for you to prosper *and be in health!*

THE ELEVATOR

Elisha Grave Otis invented the safety brake for the elevator in 1852. Although steam and hydraulic elevators had been introduced by 1850, it was Otis who first implemented a safe elevator to carry people. This invention revolutionized the multi-storied building market.

Alas, this form of vertical transportation has been abused also. The average American will not walk up one single flight of stairs unless forced to because of a lack of an elevator! How sad. And that is not even the worst of it. They will not walk *down* one flight either. And they would have gravity in their favor!

Don't misunderstand me; I'm grateful for the elevator. When I moved from my parents' house to my own apartment on the seventh floor, it saved a lot of wear and tear on my body. I can't imagine having to carry all of my belongings up seven flights of stairs. Thank God for Brother Otis!

I now look upon the elevator as another chance to exercise.

Walk instead of ride. Three, four, five flights of stairs? No problema. I walk. It compensates for our modern, technology driven society's removal, and seeming disdain, of manual labor.

I now live in a townhouse which has a two car garage. My wife's door has an electronic door opener attached to it. I refuse to put one on my door. And it's not because I'm too cheap either. It forces me to exercise my muscles by raising and lowering it. God desires for you to prosper *and be in health*!

TELEVISION, VIDEO GAMES, INTERNET

At the end of World War II American homes had 5,000 television sets in them. These sets were black and white and had five-inch screens. By 1951, the year I was born, there were 17 million sets.

My father bought our very first TV set in either 1959 or 1960. I know it was somewhere around then because I remember watching the *Howdy Doody Show*. The last episode aired on September 24, 1960.

Although I grew to love watching TV, I wasn't consumed with it pre- to early teens. And there weren't any video games or Internet back then either.

We went outside to play. I mean good old-fashioned, old school play. We played punch ball, stoop ball, tops (using bottle caps), army, navy, giant steps, and other games I just can't recall. We ran, jumped, rode our bicycles, roller skated on the sidewalk, and rode scooters (made with a wooden milk crate with a 2 by 4 and disassembled skates nailed to it). Play wasn't just confined to the outside. Inside there were the board games, marbles, and jacks. Yes, I confess. I played jacks with my sisters.

Back in those days physical education was mandatory. In grammar and high school we had to participate in gym class. We also got plenty of sunshine, fresh air (as fresh as it could be growing up in Jersey City, anyway), and exercise. Today, the only state in which physical education is mandatory from kindergarten through grade 12 is Illinois! Is this progress?

Nowadays budget cuts are removing physical education and

health classes from public schools. Video games and high definition TVs are universal substitutes for all of the outside play we baby boomers used to engage in. The overuse of these digital wonders is causing our youth to develop severe medical problems. They are no longer engaged in good physical exercise on a daily basis. Instead of having lean, strong, and muscular bodies, our young people are carrying excessive amounts of body fat.

Overweight and obese young people are reaching epidemic proportions in the United States, and around the world. A report was issued in May of 2004 by the International Obesity Task Force of the World Health Organization (WHO). This report found that some of the factors which contributed to obesity are:

1. Increased use of motorized transportation (cars, buses)
2. A decrease in physical activity
3. More sedentary recreation (video games, TV)
4. Multiple TV channels 24/7
5. Great increase of energy dense food (junk food)
6. Increasing numbers of fast food franchises and restaurants
7. Larger food portions
8. Increased consumption of soda

The overweight and obesity epidemic is leading to an increase of type 2 diabetes in young people. Some complications of type 2 diabetes are heart disease, blindness, and nerve and kidney damage. This was unheard of when I was growing up. Unfortunately the situation is, like parent(s) like children. Parents are severely shortchanging their children. Overweight and obese parents produce overweight and obese children.

One of the Ten Commandments is *thou shalt not kill*. Many think that only means killing someone else. It, however, refers to suicide also. We are on the slow path to self-destruction (suicide). Americans are slowly and methodically committing suicide by withholding exercise from their bodies, and then stuffing it full of poison (junk food, sodas, and prescription drugs). And not only are we suffering, but our children are suffering too.

Playing endless hours of video games doesn't benefit anyone

either, except the game makers (biiigggg profits). And the only body part that is exercised by Microsoft's Xbox 360 and Nintendo is the thumbs. Endless hours of mind-numbing television are not any better. Not when it replaces outdoor physical activity. And with TV, not even the thumbs are exercised.

In a year, the average child spends 900 hours in school and nearly 1,023 hours in front of a TV. This statistic is appalling.

". . . According to the American Academy of Pediatrics (AAP), kids in the United States watch about 4 hours of TV a day - even though the AAP guidelines say children older than 2 should watch no more than 1 to 2 hours a day of quality programming. . . "[12]

It has been shown through studies that children who spend more than 4 hours watching TV on a daily basis are likely to be overweight. They are physically inactive and have a tendency to snack on junk food (empty calories). They are also exposed to commercials about junk foods such as potato chips and soda. When they have finished playing the video games and watching TV, what do our young people have to occupy their time? The internet! Growing up in this day and age has turned into a curse. But growing up in the 50s and 60s there were no video games and no internet, and a minimum of TV watching (that is, when a household finally got one).

My father was a preacher. In place of TV, video games, and the internet were outdoor play, discipline, and Bible lessons. And my father was health conscious. One of the stores that he frequented was the health food store. And one of the products that he bought at that store was wheat germ. Unlike many parents today, my father wasn't stingy. He shared the wheat germ with us (that's a nice way of saying that he made us sprinkle it on our food!).

My father probably wasn't aware of it but he planted the seeds to obeying God's command to Adam, and to his progeny. Take care (manage) the earth and everything on it. That includes man's body, which came directly from the earth. Everything that God has made deserves the utmost care and respect.

Parents, the Bible says, "Train up a child in the way he should go: and when he is old, he will not depart from it" (Proverbs

22:6). The training is for the complete person. Teach the children about God and His love for us and His plan of salvation, and teach them about caring for their bodies, which He so lovingly gave us.

Television and the internet do have redeeming values. When used in moderation, TV can be used to entertain and relax, and to learn. The internet has much more value. It is a virtual repository of information. I love to read and research. In the days before the invention of the internet, the library was my ultimate source of information. I made extensive use of it. Now I can get that same information on the internet. I don't have to leave home.

The internet, too, has been abused. There are people who literally spend hours upon hours "surfing." This time can be used more productively by exercising, Bible reading and studying, enjoying the family, etc. God desires for you to prosper *and be in health!*

ESCALATOR

The escalator is an off-shoot of the elevator. A man by the name of Jesse Reno obtained a patent for a device consisting of "moving stairs," or inclined elevator, on March 15, 1892. It was redesigned in 1897 by Charles Seeberger to what we see today. Part of the word 'escalator' comes from the Latin word *scala*, which means "steps."

Today escalators are found in large department stores and airports. It always amuses me when I go to the airport to see the number of people who take the escalator versus those who take the stairs. I get a lonely feeling when I walk up and down those stairs!

Escalators are a great technological invention, but again, they are overused. People deprive themselves of the benefit of the exercise of walking by always using them.

Inclined or angled escalators are bad enough. But have you ever noticed the horizontal escalators at the airports? People will opt to take them rather than walking! Unbelievable! And we wonder why health insurance is "escalating" (no pun intended), and overweight and obese individuals have become the norm rather than the exception.

God did not give us bodies to abuse this way. This is poor management. It is not good stewardship. And the worst part is, when we reap the consequences of the abuse of our bodies, whom do we blame? The devil, that's whom. I don't like the devil anymore than you do. But when it comes to poor physical health due to poor eating habits and lack of exercise, it is not the devil's fault.

My father once told me a story about the devil. He said a man walking along saw the devil sitting on the side of the road crying. The man asked the devil why he was crying. The devil replied that *everybody* blamed *everything* on him! As Christians we can't blame Satan for any medical problem resulting from our poor eating habits, and always finding excuses why not to exercise. God desires for you to prosper *and be in health!*

AIR POLLUTION

Today's society has seen more manufacturing industries than ever before. And as a result there is more air pollution than ever before. Every time we breathe we inhale a lungful of these toxins. Smoke from our chemical and petroleum plants, as well as the exhaust from cars, trucks, and buses, are poisoning our bodies.

One type of outdoor air pollution that has been receiving a lot of media attention recently is the "greenhouse effect" (also known as global warming). This is caused by the accumulation of carbon dioxide in the atmosphere. Carbon dioxide is produced when fuels are burned.

Global warming was not a problem in years past because there existed enough plants in the world to convert the carbon dioxide into oxygen. However, deforestation and other plant losses have reduced the number of plants worldwide. (God designed plants to take in carbon dioxide, convert it into oxygen, and release it into the air.) Plus, the pollution-producing technological inventions and manufacturing plants we have today did not exist in the past.

Smog and acid rain, which plague our cities, are caused by chemical reactions between sulfur dioxide, carbon monoxide, nitrogen oxide, and chemical vapors. This pollution irritates our eyes and enters the pores of the skin. Over the years we build up severe toxic levels of these chemicals in our bodies.

The long-term effects of this outdoor pollution are respiratory diseases, heart disease, and lung cancer. Of all the killers in America today, heart disease is number one. The short-term effects of pollution are bronchitis, pneumonia, headaches, nausea, and allergic reactions. People with asthma or emphysema can have their conditions aggravated by these toxic pollutants.

We also have to be concerned with indoor pollution. Cigarette smoke, the smoke from cooking and heating appliances, paints, and other household items produce health-threatening vapors. One study has found that indoor pollution can be greater than outdoor pollution. (Indoor pollutants can be 25 to 100 times greater than outdoor pollutants!)

When a pollutant is released indoors it is 1000 times likelier to reach a person's lungs than if it were released outdoors. We just can't seem to win for losing. It is imperative that we change our lifestyles if we are to enjoy the fullness of physical life that God intended for us on this planet!

Did you know that:

1. Americans spend about 90% of their time indoors?
2. Pollutants from cleaning and personal care products are 3 times as likely to cause cancer than outdoor pollution?
3. American homes contain approximately 1,500 hazardous substances?
4. Tobacco smoke contain about 4,000 chemicals of which 200 are known poisons such as formaldehyde and carbon monoxide; it also has about 43 carcinogens?
5. About 50% of all sicknesses are caused or aggravated by indoor pollution?

As with anything else, the people who suffer the most are those whose bodies are least able to fight pollution—the very young and the elderly!

Since it is not feasible to walk around all day with gas masks, we must equip our bodies to maximize their efforts to neutralize air pollution. This can only be done by building up the immune system. Exercise to strengthen the body and eating plenty of fruits and vegetables to get the various antioxidants is the only way. We must adopt a much healthier nutrition program than we currently have in order to successfully fight the unfortunate consequences of modern technology.

Adam, Abraham, Moses, David and the other patriarchs, as well as the early New Testament church, did not have the negative impact of technology to contend with. We do. Contrary to the saying "ignorance is bliss," ignorance of the dangers of technology impacts your quality of life, and the richness that God desires for you *in the body*.

THE ELECTRIC DOOR

They are everywhere. In airports, in malls and supermarkets, and at big name franchises such as Best Buy, Circuit City, Staples, Home Depot, etc. It is an invention which takes away our getting to exercise our upper bodies during the course of everyday activities. It is the electric door.

Some electric doors swing open while others slide open. But however they open, they deprive us of the opportunity of exercising our upper bodies. I know that some of you are really broken up about that. If you really think about it though, this was the only exercise we got for our upper bodies without specifically targeting it through weight lifting. Back in the day when walking was in style and there were no electric doors, at least we got to exercise our lower and upper bodies without going to the gym.

I know electric doors are signs of progress. I also know that they are very convenient. But I think the disadvantages outweigh the overall benefit to the body as far as fitness is concerned. It wouldn't be as bad that if for every electric door there were at least one ordinary manual door. At least there would be a choice.

I know that since I brought this to your attention through this book you will be looking for manual doors to go through (yeah, right).

Even for health and fitness conscious individuals like me, entering through electric doors is the only way we will ever go in. By now it is second nature. They have been around too long.

A few stores have manual and electric doors. Sad to say, even at those stores which have both forms of doors, the electric ones are the only doors ever used. Even if a bottleneck was to occur at the electric doors, I don't think that anyone would bother using the manual ones. If I don't catch myself, I, too, will ignore the manual doors. But then again, I do exercise four days a week at the gym.

As for its history, the automatic sliding door was invented in 1954 by Lew Hewitt and Dee Horton. The first one was installed in 1960. It was operated by a mat actuator rather than by breaking a light beam. The idea came to them when they saw how the high winds in Corpus Christi, Texas, made the operation of swing doors very difficult.

MISCELLANEOUS

Let's not forget about the household labor-saving devices that have reduced or eliminated manual effort. When I was growing up, my mother washed our clothes in the bathtub with a scrub board. We didn't have an electric washing machine. We also didn't have a vacuum cleaner. Actually, we didn't need one because our floors were either linoleum or wood (and I'm not talking about good, expensive hardwood either).

Neither were there any electric dishwashers or dryers. Our dryer was a clothes line on the roof, and my mother had to carry the clothes up a flight of stairs to get to the roof! How many could do that today without "huffin" and "puffin"? Or worse yet, how many could do it without having a cardiac arrest? What a disaster!

We opened tin cans with a good old-fashioned can opener. That was really great for the arms. There were no "pop" tops back then. Remember the automobile before electric windows were installed in them? We exercised our arms another way—by cranking the windows up and down.

Before the gasoline-powered snow blowers and lawn mowers, we shoveled snow and pushed mowers through grass and weed. Face it—our parents and grandparents were fitter than we are. A lot of young people today wouldn't have been able to keep up with my father if he were alive today. He passed away at the age of 87, fit, healthy, and active.

There is nothing wrong with technological inventions. They save a lot of time, and remove drudgery from the home. But we do need to replace the fitness-generating activities that these machines eliminated, with exercise.

They call these devices *labor-saving* for a reason. The result of their saving you physical labor is more time at your disposal. That time should be used to implement a good exercise routine. An unfit body is just like a car that has never been given a tune-up. It becomes less efficient, less reliable, and in the long run will wear out faster and cost more to repair.

A fit and healthy body will reward you handsomely. You will wake up in the morning ready, willing, and able to tackle any problem you encounter. You will be better able to handle stress, and not have it cause a physical problem. You will not believe how great you will feel. There will be no aches or pains. Your muscles will be toned and primed—ready to move mountains if need be (I exaggerate but you get the point). You also will be able to impress your boss by qualifying for a good attendance certificate year after year (you can use that to remind him come review time).

How do I know all this? Because I am experiencing it right now. My body is fit and healthy. It is fit from exercise and healthy by my not taking prescription and nonprescription drugs and by eating nutritious, heart-healthy meals (junk food only occasionally). Most people don't know what it is to have a properly functioning body. They are under the wrong impression that as one gets older, one's body is supposed to become fragile, and subject to all manner of ailments. Nothing could be further from the truth. Implementing God's maintenance plan and a little common sense will prevent that.

An unhealthy body as a result of advancing years is not God's plan, and it shouldn't be yours. I don't subscribe to that old wives' tale, and you shouldn't either. Proverbs 23:7a says, "For as he thinketh in his heart, so is he. . . ." Our minds need to be transformed from Satan's lie concerning the physical body to God's truth. Remember God's word in III John 2. "Beloved, I wish above all things that thou mayest prosper and be in health, even as thy soul prospereth."

TIME

Are you surprised that I have included "time" in this chapter? Well think about it. So much more has been added to our plates in the last couple of decades that families do not take the time anymore to prepare and eat healthy meals. You would think that with the advent of the many labor-saving devices, and burgeoning technology, we would have much more leisure time. Unfortunately the exact opposite has happened. We have less leisure time.

I remember when I was growing up that not only did we eat nutritious meals, we, a family of twelve, ate *together*. That seems unbelievable nowadays. My mother did not have to try to squeeze cooking in between her full-time job because her full-time job was taking care of the house and us.

Today each member of the household has a hectic schedule and his or her own agenda. We're so busy running between school activities, meetings, practices, work, and, factoring in the commute time to get to these activities, we don't have time to sit down and eat a healthy meal together. So what do we do? We grab a saturated fat-laden burger and an order of over-salted french fries with a super-sized, sugar-filled Coke to wash it all down with. Or we grab a snack from a vending machine. And we call that lunch. And we wonder why we along with our children are obese, feeling sluggish, and have type II diabetes!

Though I can't blame technology directly for the hectic lives we live, and its subsequent effect on eating, I do blame it indirectly. Let me explain. Because of technological innovations, there are more things to buy. Big screen, digital TVs, home theater systems, computers, cell phones, and other electronic devices which did not exist 20 to 30 years ago, are selling in increasing numbers. There is nothing inherently wrong with these gadgets. But in order to afford these things, and due to inflation, we have to work harder and longer. In most cases this includes both parents having to work.

Automation and new technology have eliminated many jobs and the people working at them. You would think that the new 21st century manufacturing plants and offices would give workers more time, and less hectic schedules. But with less workers and even better technology, those fortunate enough to keep their jobs have to do the work of the people who were victims of corporate downsizing. They are doing the jobs of two or more people. So they work longer just to keep up. And what about the people who have to work two or three jobs just to make ends meet?

With such heavy schedules, spending any amount of time in the kitchen on a daily basis just isn't possible. So oftentimes it's off to our friendly neighborhood fast food restaurant or pizza parlor. I call these places "Fat City." Or, equally as bad, we toss frozen processed food in the microwave oven. And this is the rule rather than the exception.

Neglecting to prepare nutritious meals for ourselves and for our children is not God glorifying. First of all, it is sending the wrong message to the children because this behavior will most likely be replicated when they become parents. Second of all, it is grossly disrespecting the body God has created. The neglectful eating habits are poisoning the body and causing them to self-destruct. We are living beneath our privilege and not in the way God wants us to live.

Time, or rather the lack of it, coupled with leisure technology, also prevents our youth from spending any useful amount of time in the sun. These days the medical community is sending the message that sun exposure is harmful to the body. Growing up, my summers were spent all day in the sun. I don't have skin cancer. There was a recent study in the San Francisco Bay area involving 905 men aged 40 to 79 years old. Researchers found that greater exposure to the sun reduced the risk of developing prostate cancer. Of course sun burns should be avoided. But research shows that your bare skin should be exposed to the sun for at least 20 minutes for cancer prevention. It has also been found that some of the ingredients in popular sun screen lotions are carcinogenic (cancer causing).

Another dangerous by-product of our rush, rush, rush, time-driven society is stress. Natural disasters, inner city crime, terrorist attacks, that big job presentation due to start in 10 minutes and you are running 20 minutes late, an upcoming mid-term exam, all cause stress, which can take its toll on body and mind. This is the same reaction that you would experience if you were trying to escape a rampaging Black Bear. This is called the "flight-or-fight" syndrome.

> "Your pituitary gland. . . steps up its release of adrenocorticotropic hormone (SCTH), which signals other glands to produce additional hormones. . . this alarm tells your adrenal glands. . . to release a flood of stress hormones into your bloodstream. These hormones— including cortisol and adrenaline—focus your concentration, speed your reaction time, and increase your strength and agility. . ."[13]

When the circumstance that produced the stress is no longer a threat, the high levels of cortisol and adrenaline in the bloodstream return to normal. Your rapidly pounding heart and elevated blood pressure resume their regular pace. If, however, stressful situations happen multiple times back to back, your body doesn't have a chance to recover. And what is the result? Your body is thrown out of "kilter." You are at an increased risk for heart disease, insomnia, obesity, depression, and digestive system problems.

The stress brought about by current events, the pressures that arise from attempting to juggle time between family and job, and the ever changing economic climate can be handled by doing one of two things. We can "chuck" the technological rat-race, gather the family together and move to the Himalayan Mountains of northern Pakistan and join the Hunzas. Or, we can sufficiently build our bodies and nourish and maintain them in order to efficiently handle stress. For most of us, the first choice is not an option.

One of the methods to better enable the body to diffuse the negative effects of stress is to take care of it. Three things are paramount in accomplishing this task:

1. Getting enough sleep
2. Proper nutrition
3. Physical exercise

It should also go without saying that a positive mental outlook and a minimum of worry will go a long way, too.

There is no way around it. If the body is not strong enough to handle the damaging effects of stress, and if there is no outlet for the buildup of nervous energy, physical symptoms will result. These symptoms consist of, but are not limited to, asthma, vulnerability to colds, the flu, etc. because of a weakened immune system, stomach aches or diarrhea, depression, loss of appetite and/or sex drive, heart disease, and stroke.

CONVENIENCE

"... The US obesity problem has particular resonance, perhaps because it is a reflection of the modern way of life the country typifies, with its junk food and technology of convenience..."[14]

Let's face it; we have become lazy, soft, and complacent in this modern age. And as a result our health suffers. We are striving for academic excellence, financial freedom, and job and political equality while allowing the foundation of the body to rot away. A strong mind in a weak body is just not going to work. (This is a restatement of the phrase *a sound mind in a sound body* written by the English philosopher John Locke [1632–1704]). You cannot enjoy financial independence or academic excellence when you are constantly being hospitalized or at are home sick as a result of neglecting your body.

Although I consider this sub-topic to be closely associated with the previous sub-topic, *Time,* I also think that it is so important as to warrant a separate in-depth analysis. As with anything else, "convenience" can be taken to the extreme. I think that our rapidly advancing technology has lulled us into doing just that. This is especially true in America.

If you want to introduce any concept, idea, law, or change in general, to any group, it can be accomplished with a 100% success rate through a program of *gradualism.* An example of this process is the question of security. At first, closed circuit cameras appeared in department stores, and then slowly they began to appear in convenience stores, banks, and post offices. This hasn't happened all at once, but slowly—gradually. Now we have become so accustomed to them that we don't even notice or pay attention to them. I'm not judging whether they are taking away our individual freedom or not, but just giving an example so that you will better understand what will follow.

The process of gradualism has come along on the back of advancing technology. The end result of gradualism is "convenience." All across the nation stores such as Krauszer's, Quick Chek, 7-Eleven, and others just like them have popped up over the years. These stores are called *convenience* stores. And a new trend has come on the scene. There are convenience-like stores located at gas stations. Some are called *food-marts* or *quick marts.*

Since convenience stores are ubiquitous, we tend to patronize them quite often. "What's the harm?" you may be asking. Glad you asked. Look at the items in these stores. Potato chips of all varieties and descriptions, pretzels, candies, sodas, chewing gums galore, and pastries comprise the bulk of the items sold at these stores. Sandwiches can also be purchased at most of them. All of these items can be summarized in two words—junk food. At least in the typical supermarket there is a section, albeit small, containing organic foods.

The typical American diet consists of junk food. That coupled with a nonexistent exercise program presents a problem. This is why I described Americans as "lazy" and soft" at the beginning of this section. The proliferation of convenience stores and mini-marts just makes a bad situation worse. The greater the availability and the more convenient the store, the more they will be patronized.

I had a sweet tooth when I was growing up. (Truth be told, I still have that sweet tooth.) I ate lots of ice cream, pastries and candies. But at least breakfast, lunch, and dinner were solid, home-cooked and prepared meals. That's not true today. Most of our jobs and schools contain vending machines filled with junk food and sodas. These are our snacks. Our lunches are bought from McDonald's or Burger King or the many other fast food stores. And our breakfast, if eaten at all, the single most important meal of the day, is purchased from Dunkin' Donuts. None of this processed food will lead to good health.

Convenience promotes neither fitness nor health. When I was growing up it was rare to see an overweight child. My friends and classmates and I were "lean and mean." We were fit and healthy. Being overweight or obese was the exception, not the rule. Today there has been a 180 degree shift. Overweight and obesity in the young is the rule rather than the exception. Look at the children going to and from school. A great number of them are extraordinarily heavy. And I am talking about elementary school youngsters as well as high schoolers. The harm brought about by convenience has become a national epidemic. When we come to regard being overweight and obese as the norm, and think that there is something wrong with a normal, healthy weight (thin and slender), it means that the epidemic has existed for too long. Convenience stores have made our lives a little too convenient.

I remember once having a conversation at the gym with a person who had lost a significant amount of weight through diet and exercise. He was telling me that his acquaintances were now telling him that he had lost too much weight and that he was too thin. Their minds were so conditioned by time by seeing so many overweight and obese individuals, that when they saw someone with a healthy and normal body weight who was once overweight, it looked to them like he was anorexic.

Bulging stomachs and ever expanding waistlines are not a sign of a healthy weight. A friend of mine went to Wal-Mart recently to buy some work pants. He had to ask a salesperson if there were any 32 inch waist pants in stock. The smallest he saw displayed were 38 inch! What a sad commentary. There is a crisis in America.

NON-STICK COOKWARE

Just when you thought it was safe to go back into the water, I haven't finished yet with the negative health effects of technology. There is another modern convenience which, though not detracting from physical exercise as much as the preceding innovations, does impact the health. This modern technological convenience is Teflon. Teflon cookware coating made our lives easier by not allowing food to stick to the pan's surface. As a consequence, millions of housewives were deprived of exercising their arm and shoulder muscles by scrubbing hard, caked on food particles. I know the housewives reading this are mad about that.

Teflon was invented at the Dupont plant by Dr. Roy Plunkett on April 6, 1938. Obviously it has been around for awhile. What Dr. Plunkett didn't realize was that when Teflon is heated to high temperatures, it releases a toxic gas that can cause serious health problems to those exposed to it. This problem is not restricted to Teflon either. Any non-stick coating can cause a similar problem.

The Environmental Protection Agency has targeted a specific chemical used to manufacture Teflon as the culprit. The chemical, perfluorooctanic acid (PFOA) and its salts, have been found to create a potential risk of developmental and other adverse effects. The EPA's research of this chemical in laboratory rats found that PFOA may be carcinogenic (cancer-causing) also.

As seems to be standard procedure when a company's biggest money-maker is suspected of causing health issues, Dupont did not see fit to alert the millions of customers who purchased

Teflon coated cookware. Dupont in effect hid the problem by remaining "mum" about it. Because of DuPont's foot-dragging, more than 24 lawyers representing 73 people in 15 states met in Des Moines, Iowa, to put together a consumer class action suit against Dupont. Lawsuits currently on file tell how toxic gases are released when cookware coated with Teflon reached temperatures of 464 degrees or higher. The fumes have been found to kill pet birds kept in kitchens in which there is no ventilation, as well as cause cancer in laboratory animals.

There is an easy solution to cleaning regular cookware. Allow it to soak in water for a few minutes and then either sponge it away, or use a brillo pad. Water is very corrosive and given time will dissolve almost anything. Due to health concerns, I recommend tossing away all Teflon coated cookware and using regular pots and pans. This way you eliminate one of the health risks that will interfere with you living a God-glorifying life through good health. And by applying a little "elbow grease," you get to exercise those arm and shoulder muscles.

CHAPTER 3:

Television Commercials and Declining Health

INTRODUCTION

My father was a strict holiness preacher. We weren't allowed to go to the movies, parties, or watch certain programs on TV. And forget about having girlfriends and boyfriends at the age children today are having them. Of course my father didn't believe in smoking or drinking either. Whenever a cigarette or any alcoholic beverage commercial came on TV, we had to get up and turn down the volume until it was over. I know you're laughing right about now. But then it was a pain in the neck. Here we were, all comfortable, enjoying the program. And then a cigarette commercial pops up. And we had better not "dilly dally" in getting to the set either (we did not have a remote control). The only programs we were allowed to watch were family oriented shows. Some of my favorites were *Lassie*, *Dennis the Menace*, and *My Favorite Martian*. My father purchased a television in the early days before cigarette commercials were banned.

I don't think my father fully realized the implications of his actions. Cigarettes and alcoholic beverages are harmful to the body and we were not allowed to be indoctrinated by that garbage. Only within the last few years have we (the general public) realized how deadly cigarette smoking is.

Last chapter we looked at the television set itself and how it is abused. In this chapter we will discover how the commercials that are shown during the course of normal programming are sabotaging our bodies' health.

Television is a very powerful medium through which to proclaim a message. It adds the dimension of sight to the sound of its enormously popular predecessor, the radio. Coupling images to audio messages enables the advertising industry to propagate any message they desire, and have it sear itself deep into the viewer's mind. The viewer becomes programmed in a sense. It's like a person who has been hypnotized and given a post-hypnotic suggestion. Upon being awakened from the hypnotic state, he feels compelled to perform the suggestion.

Through the Saturday morning cartoon and children's programs' time slots, advertisers are using powerful imagery to seduce powerless youngsters. The ubiquitous clown Ronald McDonald is the carrot on the stick to plant McDonald's restaurant into children's minds. Once at the restaurant, children have a colorful, plastic play area, and toys galore. They are loyal future consumers in the making.

America's sickness industry (it masquerades under the name of healthcare system) costs us over $1 trillion per year. This industry is fueled in a large part through television advertising. Think about this. The majority of the commercials on TV concern either prescription drugs or processed food (including soft drinks). Why is America self-destructing? Because of the health crisis that is generated in a large part by prescription and nonprescription drugs and processed food. The other reason America's health is failing is due to lack of exercise.

PRESCRIPTION AND
NONPRESCRIPTION DRUGS

In the early 1990s Dr. Jeffrey Wigand exposed the hidden secrets of the tobacco industry. Back then it was a 50 billion dollar a year business. Dr. Wigand had been hired by the Brown & Williamson Tobacco Company to find a safer cigarette. Brown & Williamson was the third largest cigarette company behind Philip Morris and R. J. Reynolds. Dr. Wigand's testimony revealed that the CEOs of the major tobacco companies lied to Congress when they testified that they did not know of the addictive nature of nicotine. As a matter of fact, addictiveness was their objective. Cigarettes were a delivery device for nicotine. The story of Dr. Wigand and Big Tobacco was dramatized in a movie named *The Insider* (1999). Russell Crowe portrayed Dr. Jeffrey Wigand. Big Tobacco was driven by one motive and one motive only—the profit motive! Remember I Timothy 6:10. "For the love of money is the root of all evil: which while some coveted after, they have erred from the faith, and pierced themselves through with many sorrows."

The 21st century is seeing the same thing as the 90s. Only this time it is the pharmaceutical companies who are the culprits. The drug industry is a multi-billion dollar industry. I think this industry is worse than Big Tobacco because we are conditioned to believe that prescription and nonprescription drugs are not only necessary, but that there is no alternative.

Why do I compare the pharmaceutical industry with the tobacco industry of the early 90s? Because the pharmaceutical industry like the tobacco industry, is profit driven. They know the dangers of their drugs just like the tobacco industry knew the dangers of nicotine. They just don't care about your health. The pharmaceutical industry doesn't want to find cures for *any* health problem. A cure would erode away their enormous profits.

I might as well tell you from the outset that I don't believe in drugs (those synthetic products made by the pharmaceutical industry). I believe that if you do develop some medical condition, there are natural remedies which can be used as alternatives. These natural remedies are plants and herbs and their by-products which God has provided all over the earth. He has given us everything needed for good health.

And since these natural remedies created by God on the third day (Read Genesis 1:11–13), are all natural, they do not produce any side effects. The body sees all pharmaceutical drugs as invaders. The body attempts to fight off these invaders and the results are the side effects which sometimes are as bad as, or even worse, than the condition for which the drug was originally taken.

Many a time my father would tell me that when he was growing up (he was born in 1898) his parents would go into the woods looking for herbs and roots if any of them got sick. I'm sure many of you reading this have heard similar stories. They didn't go to the drugstore for an 'over the counter' drug. Neither did they go to Dr. So and So's office to get a prescription.

I consider myself to be truly blessed. I can say without hesitation that with exercise and a healthy diet, and avoiding prescription and nonprescription drugs, you can live a pain and illness free life. I don't now, and have never in my life taken any prescription or nonprescription drug. I did take aspirin though on a couple of occasions decades ago. But other than that time, I have taken nothing. I also refuse to get flu shots.

And what are the results of my depriving the pharmaceutical industry of my money? I have never stayed overnight in any hospital. I don't get colds or the flu. I don't get headaches or stomach aches. I also don't wake up in the morning feeling "blah" or with aches and pains. I have never had a broken bone or an operation. I am not bragging and I give God the glory. But this is the type of life God wants for you, a quality life full of energy, and pain free. *This can be you!*

I should also mention that when I worked for Elizabethtown Gas Company, I received a certificate for perfect attendance every year that they offered it. I don't get sick so I couldn't justify staying home. Also in my almost thirty-one years with the gas company, I have never had to take advantage of their prescription drug program. I carried a prescription drug card around with me, but never had to use it.

This can be you. Think of how much money you could save

on doctor visits and prescriptions if you would just implement an exercise program and good eating habits into your life. Think of how much you could accomplish in your ministry and job or business if you weren't hindered by sickness, lack of energy, doctor visits, and hospital stays!

I remember something my chemistry teacher told my class back in high school. He said, "A word to the wise is sufficient." I have always remembered that because I consider it sound advice. When I read books and articles about the dangers of prescription and nonprescription drugs, and what God's Word says about my body, and the care and respect I should give it, I implemented those principles.

Let's go again to Genesis 1:29. "And God said, Behold, I have given you every herb bearing seed, which is upon the face of all the earth, and every tree, in the which is the fruit of a tree yielding seed; to you it shall be for meat."

God knows exactly what nutrients the human body needs for optimum health and vitality. He placed them on the earth *before* he put man on it. Man is God's creation and is therefore limited. It is impossible for him to devise 'better' processes and invent alternate but equal foods. Man thinks that he knows more than his Creator, but he doesn't. It's the devil's lie. The devil told Eve that if she ate of the fruit of the tree which stood in the middle of the garden, she would be as God (Genesis 3:1–5). Ever since man has been deluded that he is God's equal or superior.

The problem that pharmaceutical companies have with herbs and roots (the alternative remedies created by God) is that they cannot be patented. This means that the pharmaceutical industry cannot have exclusive rights to them and make obscene amounts of profit. The only way for them to make money is to formulate synthetic drugs from chemicals, and then apply for a patent. Once approved by the FDA (Food and Drug Administration), they can market their "wonder" drug and make lots of *moolah*!

While watching the news this evening, a drug called Aricept was advertised. This drug, which is manufactured by the pharmaceutical company Pfizer, is for people who have mild to moderate Alzheimer's disease. Here is a portion of the company's disclaimer, ". . . Aricept is well tolerated but may not be for everyone. Some people may have nausea, diarrhea, not sleep well, or vomit. Some people may have muscle cramps, feel very tired, or may not want to eat. . . Some people who take Aricept may experience fainting. . . "[15]

This type of disclaimer is not unique to Aricept. Every drug advertised, whether on television or in magazines, has a similar disclaimer.

What you won't see advertised in the media is that German scientists have discovered a natural substance found in every cell of the human body which halts the progression of Alzheimer's disease. It's called alpha lipoic acid. Researchers have known for years that alpha lipoic acid can assist in the slowing down of the aging process. But what these German researchers have done is to increase the dosage. They gave people who had been diagnosed with Alzheimer's disease a dosage of 600 milligrams a day of alpha lipoic acid. This group was monitored for a year. Every person given this dosage had the progress of the disease halted dead in its tracks. There was no further loss of brain power. The only thing is that mega doses of this substance can reduce the level of biotin in the body. To prevent that from happening, a person need only take 300 micrograms of biotin with the 600 milligrams of alpha lipoic acid.

My mother was diagnosed with Alzheimer's disease. When I found this information in an alternative medicine piece of literature, I immediately went to the Vitamin Shoppe and bought alpha lipoic acid and biotin. I told my mother about this and had her stop taking the prescription drug she had been given by her doctor, and begin taking the natural (God created) combination with her dinner.

There are no disclaimers with alpha lipoic acid because there are no side effects, serious or otherwise. When you stick to God's herbs and plants which he specifically designed for man's benefit and use, there will be no side effects.

Pfizer doesn't want the general public to know about this Alzheimer's disease remedy, or any other natural cure, because they can't patent it. And since they can't patent it, they can't have exclusive rights to manufacture and sell it. When there aren't exclusive rights to a product, enormous profits cannot be generated.

I take alpha lipoic acid myself. Although I haven't been diagnosed with Alzheimer's disease, I find the benefits too good to pass up. Even if I was in the process of getting Alzheimer's, the fact that I am taking this natural substance will prevent it from getting worse. In addition to stopping the progression of Alzheimer's disease, alpha lipoic acid helps fight the aging process.

The cigarette and cigar commercials of yesteryear have been replaced by drug commercials. Only the drug commercials are a lot more sophisticated. They are well thought out by Madison Avenue advertising agencies. And they all seem so sincere. You would honestly think that the pharmaceutical companies have your best interests at heart. *They do not!* These pharmaceutical companies budget literally billions of dollars on advertising.

> . . . In 2000, pharmaceutical companies spent $2.5 billion on mass media pharmaceutical advertisements, according to Mike Fillon in *Ephedra: Fact or Fiction.* This number increased to over $3 billion in 2003, according to Dr. John Abramson's book *Overdosed America.* . . [16]

> . . . These days, it's hard to tell the difference between pharmaceutical commercials and car commercials. Both are almost always intended to look 'cool.' Car and pharmaceutical commercials use the same hooks—popular music, good acting and lofty promises—to hook consumers and reel them in. . . [17]

Contrary to the claims in commercials and in newsprint, drug companies are not searching for cures for high cholesterol, diabetes, Alzheimer's disease, cancer, or any other medical condition. A cure for any medical condition would mean a loss of patients. Patients no longer requiring medication would represent a loss of enormous profits. To give you an idea of the amount of money involved in pharmaceutical drugs, the March 30, 2006 edition of the *The Star-Ledger* ran an article entitled *A Hole in the Market*.

The article concerned the fact that Merck's number 2 selling cholesterol lowering drug (also known as a statin), Zocor, loses its patent in June. (The number 1 selling cholesterol lowering drug in the world is Lipitor which is manufactured by Pfizer). That means that any pharmaceutical company could produce generic brands of the drug Zocor—inexpensive generic brands. The cholesterol lowering drug market alone is worth $16 billion. Other top patents due to expire in 2006 are:

Zocor- statin (Merck), sales: $3.1 billion
Zoloft- depression (Pfizer), sales: $2.6 billion
Ambien- sleep aid (Sanofi-Aventis), sales: $1.5 billion
Pravachol- statin (Bristol-Myers Squibb), sales: $1.3 billion
Zofran- antiemetic (GlaxoSmithKline), sales: $1 billion.

Top patents due to expire in 2007 are:

Norvasc- blood pressure (Pfizer), sales: $2.2 billion
Risperdal- antipsychotic (Johnson & Johnson), sales: $1.9 billion
Zyrtec- allergy (Pfizer), sales: $1.4 billion
Lotrel- blood pressure (Novartis), sales: $1.1 billion

These are United States sales figures from 2005.

All of the above sales figures are at least one billion dollars. (Think about it, 1 billion equals 1,000 million!) This listing is only a small sampling of the drugs being produced, and represents a fraction of the total drug market. The pharmaceutical companies are making huge profits from the average American.

Every legitimate business, no matter what it is, has a right to make a profit. The food industry and the pharmaceutical industry are no exceptions. In order for a manufacturing company to make a profit, it has a right to markup its price. But ethically speaking, the markup should be reasonable. The markups by Big Pharma are obscene. For instance let's take a look at the drug Lipitor which is manufactured by Pfizer. It costs Pfizer $5.80 to manufacture 20 mg (milligrams) of Lipitor. They charge the patient $272! If you think that's bad, let's take a look at Prozac which is manufactured by Eli Lilly and company. It costs them 11 cents to make 20 mg of this drug. Prozac however is sold for $247! Not only are these synthetic drugs dangerous, but you are charged a ridiculous amount for something that is harmful to you.

Today's *Star-Ledger* carried a front page story concerning the pharmaceutical company Merck. "A state court jury ruled that Merck failed to warn two Vioxx patients about the risks of the drug and held the Whitehouse Station-based company liable for the heart attack suffered by one of the plaintiffs, awarding him and his wife $4.5 million. . . " (Thursday, April 6, 2006).

A panel also found Merck guilty of fraud by intentionally misrepresenting Vioxx's cardiovascular risks, and leaving out or hiding important information from doctors.

Big Pharma (the pharmaceutical industry) has advertisements for the entire range of physical and medical problems. There are prescription and OTC (over the counter) drugs targeted at sleeplessness, erectile dysfunction (notably Viagra), high blood pressure, Alzheimer's disease, high cholesterol, acid reflux, heartburn, osteoporosis, ad infinitum!

> To make matters worse, though, the general public has been brainwashed by TV ads, the news media, and the FDA into believing that prescription drugs enrich their lives. Many also still believe that government agencies such as the FDA ensure that these drugs are safe and perform the way the pharmaceutical companies claim they do. Hogwash.[18]

FAST AND PROCESSED FOOD

> . . . A 1991 study showed that there was an average of 200 junk food ads in 4 hours of children's Saturday morning cartoons. . . [19]

> . . . Studies have shown that a typical child is exposed to 40,000 candy, cereal, soda and fast food ads a year and several food marketing campaigns are using children's favorite television and movie characters such as SpongeBob Cheez, Scooby-Doo cereals and Teletubbies Happy Meals. In many cases this exposure determines the kinds of foods the child will pick out or request in grocery stores. . . [20]

These facts are appalling but not surprising. Target young, impressionable minds with appealing food commercials and build a lifetime customer. Taste is one of the strongest senses we possess. Junk food appeals to the taste buds and the consumer becomes literally addicted to the taste. And, like drug addicts, they have to have their daily "fix." When they become adults and have children, they too will feed their children the same types of good tasting, fattening, and artery clogging empty calories.

While watching CNN (Cable Network News) the other day I saw another alarming story. Car seat manufacturers will have to build larger car seats because children are no longer able to fit into the standard seat. Large numbers of children are now overweight and obese. News concerning overweight and obese children, in addition to overweight and obese adults, is escalating.

> An alarming number of poor children in New York City are obese by age 2 according to a new study. . . An even larger number of toddlers are overweight. Of 16,000 city kids enrolled in the program, 40 percent are too heavy for their age. . . Frieden and Children's Services Commissioner John B. Mattingly urged parents to encourage their children to be physically active, spend less time watching television and stay away from junk food and sugary drinks. . . [21]

While working out in the gym this morning, I got into a conversation in between sets with an associate named Henry. We somehow got on the subject of the obesity epidemic. Henry told me that ten-year-old little leaguers in his town averaged 200 pounds in weight! I found that disturbing but not unbelievable. What is the cause? Too little exercise and too many empty calories.

A friend of mine and his wife told me something back in the late 70s or very early 80s. In retrospect I find it unique, and an attitude which should be more in evidence today. She said that she would abstain from eating sweets while pregnant. It took me by surprise, and unfortunately I have since forgotten what prompted it.

In those early days overweight and obese kids were not an issue. If the mother avoided sweets while carrying the child, the child would not have a craving for it when growing up. That's half the battle.

THE HISTORY OF FAST FOOD

The phrase *fast food* was originally part of the title of a trade magazine called *Fountain and Fast Food Service*. The magazine was renamed *Fast Food* in 1960. Its February issue contained the following statement: "delicate scallops are *really* fast food. . . because they come ready to cook." And in July of the same year we find this remark, "Fast food type restaurants do the lion's share of business for breakfast and noon meals eaten out."

White Castle is generally recognized as the very first fast food restaurant in America. It made its first appearance in 1921. White Castle started out by selling hamburgers for 5 cents. Needless to say White Castle has become very successful. Many competitors followed.

The world's largest fast food chain is McDonald's. It made its appearance in San Diego, California, in 1948. Ray Kroc joined McDonald's founders in 1954 and expanded the franchise. He was originally a distributor of an industrial milkshake mixer that McDonald's used. Wendy's was founded in 1972. It introduced the "drive-thru" window which is so popular today.

The "fast" in *fast food* is there for a reason. It is designed to serve the customer as quickly as possible. In order to do this, fast foods are highly processed (I view this as tampering with natural foods) with standardized ingredients, cooking and production methods.

Fast food franchises' cooking methods are especially suspect in today's accelerating obesity rates. Items such as french fries and burgers are deep fried in partially hydrogenated oils (also known as trans fats). When vegetable oils are hardened into margarine or shortening, trans fatty acids are formed. Trans fats are found in fast food staples such as french fries and fried chicken. But these fats go beyond just fast food restaurants. Processed food manufacturers use trans fats in doughnuts, cookies, crackers, pastries, cereals, and waffles. These manufacturers use trans fats because they are cheaper than oil, they extend the shelf life of the products, can be used over and over again and they are frequently used to provide flavor and texture.

Trans fatty acids are much more dangerous than the saturated fats they replaced. They have been found to increase the blood levels of low density lipoprotein cholesterol (LDL) while at the same time lowering the levels of high density lipoprotein (HDL). LDL cholesterol is the "bad" cholesterol and HDL is the "good" cholesterol. Trans fats also clog the arteries, are linked to type 2 diabetes and other serious health problems such as heart disease.

Along with high trans fat products such as french fries and fried chicken, fast food restaurants also serve high sugar content sodas. And now they don't just serve the small standard sized soda, you can choose the super-sized drinks. One meal from any one of these franchises can provide plenty of empty calories from their high fat and sugar products. These foods are engineered to taste good. Fast food franchises have succeeded because they do satisfy the palate.

On July 24, 2002, FoxNews.com reported that a New York City lawyer by the name of Samuel Hirsch filed a lawsuit on behalf of his client against McDonald's, Burger King, Wendy's and KFC. The suit claims that these fast food companies are irresponsible and deceptive in listing nutritional information on their products. And, like nicotine or illegal drugs, create an addiction, especially among the poor, and children.

The plaintiff in the lawsuit, Caesar Barber, 56 years old, unfortunately typifies the American of today. He consistently ate at these fast food restaurants four to five times a week. His poor eating habits resulted in obesity, diabetes, high cholesterol and blood pressure. These health problems caused two heart attacks. The courts ruled against the plaintiff. In March of 2004 congress passed a law which makes it illegal to sue any food company because their products are the cause of obesity.

While not commenting on the legality and/or validity of the lawsuit against the fast food companies, I know that lawsuits and court actions are not the answer. The consumer must be educated. And this education must begin with children.

Fast food restaurants are proliferating like rabbits. This is because the market is wide open. Fast food restaurants fit nicely into our time sensitive culture. We can't afford to wait for anything. This paradigm must change. Our health and lives are at stake. Also, continuing on this path will never lead to a God-glorifying life through good health.

I don't see as many television advertisements from the fast food restaurants as I did in the past. Then again it may be that the bulk of their television advertising is done on Saturday mornings to target the children. In actuality they really don't have a need to advertise as much. They are as well known by now both individually and collectively as today's leading actors and talk show hosts.

Like Big Pharma, and Big Tobacco before it, the food industry is profit driven. Enormous profits are at stake. An *educated* consumer is the only thing that will bring about change in this industry. There is an old saying that *money talks*. If the average consumer would refuse to patronize these fast food restaurants, or at least refuse to buy any artery clogging, high fat, high sugar, and high sodium (salt) food, and spend their hard earned money elsewhere, these restaurants will be forced to make substantial changes to their menus.

To be honest with you, we don't need these fast food restaurants. With their advent, family dinners have become a thing of the past. Dinners with every member of the family sitting together and not being pressured because of time constraints have gone with the wind. One of the most important things that God has established on earth among humans is the family. Meals should not only be eaten in a family setting, they should also be totally nutritious, and prepared with love. That means no processed and chemically treated food. Like the Hunza diet, our food should be completely organic.

Look at the appalling facts and statistics about the fast food industry:

a) 1 out of 4 Americans goes to a fast food restaurant every day
b) Americans spent more than $110 billion on fast food in 2000.
c) French fries are eaten more than any other vegetable in America
d) 60% of all Americans are either overweight or obese!
e) If things don't change, obesity will surpass smoking as the leading cause of preventable death in America
f) Diabetes will take 17 to 27 years off your life
g) Most nutritionists recommend not eating fast foods more than once a month

I recommend not eating fast food *at all*. It has no redeeming value. In 2004 Morgan Spurlock directed a documentary about the fast food industry in general, and McDonald's specifically. McDonald's is the world's largest fast food chain. The name of this documentary is *Super Size Me*. Morgan ate nothing but McDonald's for thirty days. He didn't exercise. During the course of this project, Morgan gained weight and became ill many times.

Super Size Me should be a wake up call to America. It should be required viewing for every parent and their children. Morgan Spurlock undertook his documentary to see what the effects would be if a person were to eat fast food exclusively for thirty days. He established a few ground rules. Within that thirty day period, he would eat nothing but McDonald's for each of three meals a day. He also had to eat everything on McDonald's menu at least once.

During the thirty day period Morgan was under the supervision of three doctors. He underwent a thorough physical examination before he began the experiment. Morgan's cholesterol, blood pressure, and all other numbers were normal. He started at a body weight of 185 ½ pounds and a body fat reading of 11% which is extremely good. At the end of the thirty day period, Morgan's cholesterol skyrocketed, his weight increased to 210 pounds and his body fat rose to 18%. Suffering liver damage and out of concern, his doctors and vegetarian girlfriend pleaded with him to get off the program.

As a part of the *Super Size Me* documentary, 100 nutritionists from around the country were interviewed on their views of fast food. 95 out of the 100 said that fast food contributed to obesity! And a little less than half said that fast food *should not be eaten at all*.

I mentioned in a previous chapter that my father was health conscious. Besides putting wheat germ on his food, he ate no bread except stone ground whole wheat bread. He used to tell me that white bread was used as paste to hang wallpaper back in his youth. White bread, like all other processed food, is created to appeal to the sight and taste buds. It has absolutely no nutritional value at all. "... White flour, as I have mentioned previously, when mixed with water, makes paste. Eating white flour makes you fat; it can also be addicting, and clogs up your digestive system..."[22]

GET THEM WHILE THEY'RE YOUNG

There is nothing in the world as impressionable and malleable as a child's mind. When a child is in his developmental years, the propaganda the mind is fed on a continuous basis will forever impact his life. The Kaiser Family Foundation did an interesting nation wide study of 1,051 parents who had children from the ages of 6 months to 6 years old. The study is named *The Media Family: Electronic Media in the lives of Infants, Toddlers, Preschoolers and Their Parents.* Although all types of electronic viewing media were involved in this study, I will concentrate on television only.

The Kaiser study found that 19 percent of children 1 year old or younger have a TV in their bedrooms; 29 percent of children 2 to 3 years old have a TV in their bedrooms and 43 percent of children ages 4 through 6 have a TV in their bedrooms. Vicky Rideout, Vice President and Director of Kaiser's Program for the Study of Entertainment Media and Health, says the following: "Parents have a tough job, and they rely on TV in particular to help make their lives more manageable. Parents use media to help them keep their kids occupied, calm them down, avoid family squabbles, and teach their kids the things parents are afraid they don't have time to teach themselves"[23]

What does the fact that children watch too much TV have to do with living a God-glorifying life through good health? Good question. Did you know that the United States and New Zealand are the only two industrialized nations in the world which allow direct to consumer prescription drug advertisements? New Zealand is looking to ban this type of advertisement, and if successful, will leave the United States as the only industrialized nation which allows direct to consumer advertising. By the time he is 10 years old, a typical American child will have watched more than 75,000 hours of TV! This equates to about 40,000 TV ads a year. The pharmaceutical industry jams many drug commercials in an hour of TV programming. Having literally grown up by being exposed to hour after hour of professionally choreographed prescription drug commercials, children will see drugs as their first option when any type of illness hits them after they reach adulthood. The slogan of the United Negro College Fund (UNCF) is *a mind is a terrible thing to waste.* You can believe that the pharmaceutical and food industries are in total agreement. And they waste no time in capitalizing on your child's mind.

Alternative therapies and treatments are not advertised via mainstream media and so the average American is not aware of them. So as far as the average American is concerned, there is no alternative to prescription drugs.

Big Pharma has so programmed and manipulated children's

minds that after they reach adulthood they will look on every health anomaly as a disease to be treated with prescription drugs. These drugs are toxic which is evidenced by their many side effects. And what about the impact 5, 10, or 20 years down the road? It seems that our youth are predestined not to live a God-glorifying life through good health. Not if the pharmaceutical industry has anything to say about it anyway!

Television mind poisoning does not end with the pharmaceutical industry. Saturday mornings are set aside for children's prime-time cartoon programming. And who do you think does the bulk of the advertising during this block of time? If you said the food industry you are correct. I am including sodas and cereals in this category.

When I was growing up I was a big consumer of cereal. I ate Cheerios, Wheaties, Cap'n Crunch, Kellogg's Frosted Flakes, and other sugar-laden junk food. Of course neither I nor my parents were aware of the empty calories I was eating. Besides Coca-Cola and Pepsi-Cola, other popular sodas being sold when I was growing up were Royal Crown Cola and Nehi. I drank these soft drinks often in the early days.

Breakfast cereals and soft drinks, along with McDonald's and Burger King, are enormously popular with today's youth. These are what children want and this is what their parents give them. Children's impressionable minds develop an addiction for these high sugars and high fat taste treats.

At one time white bread had the distinction of being the greatest source of calories in the typical American diet. Not any more. A sampling of American adults by the National Health and Nutrition Examination Survey (NHANES) produced the following startling results: (a) over 2/3 of the adults sampled said that they drank enough sodas or sweet drinks to supply them with a greater proportion of daily calories more than any other food and (2) obesity rates were greatest among those who drank sweet drinks. This survey was conducted in 1999 - 2000. Dr. Mercola comments that obesity may lower the average age of the death of children in this country so much that their parents may outlive them. This is tragic.

I acquired a severe sweet tooth in my youth. As a matter of fact I still have it. But now I control and subjugate it for the greater good of my overall health. Not only did sodas satisfy my sweet tooth when I was young, they benefited me financially too. I lived diagonally across from Lincoln High School in Jersey City. Being the industrious lad that I was, I would collect soda bottles at lunchtime from the high school students during the spring and summer months. Hey, I redeemed them for 2 cents on the bottle. Did I save the money and put it in the bank? No. I bought Drake's Ring Dings, coffee cakes, pies, Twinkies and cookies with it. Don't laugh. I told you I had a serious sweet tooth. Solomon in his wisdom said that parents are to train up their children in the way they should go (Proverbs 22:6). Children should be given very limited exposure to sweets (sodas, breakfast cereals) and fast foods. As a matter of fact, this training should begin in the womb. The mother should not have these deceptive treats at all while carrying a child.

Limited exposure to refined foods and fast foods includes viewing them on television. After birth, a child's exposure to TV should be very limited, and monitored. No child should have a TV set in the bedroom. Oh boy, I'm in trouble now. Sounds tough? Sure it does. But look at what's happening to American youth. Many are overweight and obese. They have type 2 diabetes and are on their way to developing various cancers, high blood pressure, heart disease, multiple sclerosis, sleep apnea, Alzheimer's disease, asthma and a slew of other serious medical problems. When these children go to their doctors for health problems, and surgery is not required, how do you think these doctors are going to treat them? You are right—with prescription drugs!

The food and pharmaceutical industries provide a classic example of a vicious, unending circle. The food industries introduce their loyal consumers to the pharmaceutical industry. How do they do this? By utilizing technologies which have been proven to cause, or are linked to, whether directly or indirectly, weight gain and obesity, cancer, heart diseases, etc. The technologies used are genetic food modification (Read more about this in Chapter 5), the addition of dangerous sugars and sweeteners, the stripping away of vital nutrients and using chemical bleaching agents, and injecting cows and other animals with hormones and antibiotics. Residual amounts of these harmful chemicals find their way into the human food chain. A potential drug customer is in the making.

When a health problem emerges from eating processed foods, the consumer is prescribed the appropriate pharmaceutical medication or medications. These prescription drugs merely treat the symptom, and so the suffering consumer is doomed to take these harmful drugs for life. In the meantime, he is still eating and drinking the food companies' products which made him sick in the first place. Do you see the vicious circle? Both the food and pharmaceutical industries profit big time. The exploited consumer is like the woman with the issue of blood. She went from doctor to doctor seeking help and relief. The only thing that changed was her bank account. It dropped from something to nothing while she remained sick.

God doesn't want this for you and He certainly doesn't want it for your children. We don't have to allow the food and pharmaceutical companies to profit at our expense. An educated consumer is the food and drug industries' worst nightmare. Help me put the drug companies out of business, and at the same time force the food companies to clean up their act. If you have no need for the drug companies' drugs as I don't, they will go out of business. The best way to put the pharmaceutical companies out of business is to start with the food companies. Boycott the food companies' products until they put your welfare ahead of profit. What's that you say? "You've gotta eat?" Sure you do. But not at all costs. You have an alternative. Buy only organic foods. I guarantee that if enough people do that, the food giants will get the message quickly enough. The only way you as a consumer can effect change is through financial means. Attack the pocketbook. That's the only language they understand.

A financial boycott is a highly effective way to bring about a desired result. Remember the bus boycott in Montgomery, Alabama, in 1955? Rosa Parks refused to give up her seat on December 1, 1955. On December 5, 1955, a boycott organized by Dr. Martin Luther King on the city's bus lines began. It was 100 percent effective. The bus line was hit where it hurts—in the pocketbook. The same tactic can be applied to the food industries. And this food company boycott would have a rippling effect. As more and more people refuse to buy junk and processed food, an amazing thing would begin to happen. The whole, organic food being eaten would begin to allow the body to heal itself. The body would be given the vital and healthy nutrients that God has provided. As the healing process continues, you find that synthetic prescription drugs will no longer be needed. Slowly but surely the pharmaceutical industry would see their profits shrink. It's like a 2 for 1 deal. This is one situation where a win-lose proposition is not necessarily a bad thing. You win while the money hungry food and drug industries lose.

SIZE MATTERS

America seems to have a love affair with things "super." This summer (2006) sees the release of the latest feature length movie in the Superman series, *Superman Returns*. These movies seem to do well at the box office. And even though McDonald's eliminated its super-sized fries and drinks in 2004, the super-sized food craze still remains. All you can eat and buffet style restaurants dot the American landscape to take advantage of our cravings for super portions, and take up McDonald's slack.

McDonald's may have given in to the critics' cry for healthier portion sizes, but the movie theater certainly hasn't. You are still able to satisfy that super appetite with larger than life soft drinks and popcorn. And what about the portion sizes that restaurants serve? I can almost guarantee that any restaurant that gives anything less than super-sized portions will be closing its doors in the near future due to a shrinking clientele. America has been eating enormously large portion sizes for so long that the abnormal has become the norm.

Not only are we eating toxin and hormone infected food with very little nutritional value, but we're eating huge quantities of it. America is literally eating itself to death. While we are scratching our collective heads wondering why we are sick all the time, and dying prematurely, Satan is laughing himself silly. But we can change that. God has given us common sense and a guide book that will take us through this world as well as the next. We can refuse to eat from the devil's table (processed food) and return to the Lord's table (whole, natural food). Look what David says, "Thou preparest a table before me in the presence of mine enemies: thou anointest my head with oil; my cup runneth over" (Psalms 23:5).

TELEVISION COMMERCIALS THEN AND NOW

The advertising budget for the pharmaceutical industries' direct to consumer campaign is upwards of $4.5 billion! Ever since the FDA relaxed its guidelines in 1997, television airtime has been bombarded more and more by prescription drug commercials. Before then, sales pitches were directed to doctors only. What did television viewers see before the FDA loosened its guidelines?

One thing that television viewers did not see was a plethora of prescription and OTC (over the counter) drugs. The closest that came to them were commercials for Alka-Seltzer, Dristane, or Bufferin. When I was growing up two products which could have prevented viewers from living a God-glorifying life through good health, tobacco and alcohol, were aired on a regular basis. As I mentioned earlier, when either one aired we had to turn the volume down. Back in those days Big Tobacco was king of the airwaves. Not only did they heavily advertise through television commercials, but through the movies also. All of the movie goers' favorite actors and actresses puffed their way through every theatrical release. Bogie and Bacall, James Cagney, Bette Davis, Paul Henreid, Joan Crawford and dozens of others demonstrated class and cool with every drag on their cigarettes.

Big Tobacco's cigarette and cigar commercials were imaginative and varied. Marlboro cigarette commercials told the viewer to come to Marlboro country (1960s). Winston said that its brand "tastes good like a cigarette should" (1950s). Cool and refreshing was the come on for Kools. If we wanted fine tobacco we had to smoke Lucky Strike (1948). The alcoholic commercials were predominantly wine and beer. You had Gallo wine along with Hamm's beer, Ballantine, Carling's Black Label (animated feature shows husband calling wife, Mabel, for a Black Label beer (1950s), Budweiser (1960s), Rheingold, and Colt 45 Malt Liquor (1960s) among others.

FAST FOOD RESTAURANTS ARE EVERYWHERE

The only business which can rival drug stores for sheer numbers are the fast food franchises. Everywhere you look you are bound to see the golden arches of McDonald's, castles which are white in color (White Castle), Pizza Hut, Burger King, IHOP (International House of Pancakes), and on and on. Americans are so addicted to fast foods that even though several competitors are adjacent to each other, they are still all thriving. Americans, along with the entire world, have a love affair with fast foods.

However, not only is the outside landscape literally dotted with fast food franchises, they are also located in large shopping malls and in hospitals and schools. Yes, you heard me right, they are in hospitals too. I have always understood hospitals to be bastions of health. Realistically though, money will always talk louder than health issues. Over 4,500 school systems throughout the country serve Taco Bell products. Also over 30% of public high schools offer brand name fast foods. Meanwhile government statistics show that our children are receiving a full 50% of their calories from added sugar and fat!

How many patients are hospitalized directly or indirectly because of eating the high sugar, high fat, and high salt content of these fast food franchises' products? Although many do not see a problem with fast foods being available in hospitals and schools, I do. These non-nutritious meals are relatively cheap and they taste so good. With the eyes and nose constantly assaulted with stimulating sights and smells the consumer is helpless because he is already addicted. It's like putting a fox in the henhouse and not expecting it to have the hens for breakfast, lunch and dinner.

Before my position was eliminated from Elizabethtown Gas

Company, I would always "brown bag" it. The company did provide an outside food service to run the cafeteria, but you can never tell how the food is prepared and what is being used. Even in high school I wouldn't eat cafeteria food. I went home for lunch. Due to rapidly advancing technology which has thoroughly impacted the entire food industry, we have no choice but to eat only home-prepared organic food.

Although I never ate fast foods every day, I did eat my share of it. And now that I have given it up (I haven't had it for well over a year now) I can honestly say that I don't miss it. When I ate it I did at times have cravings for it. I have no such cravings now. Now I see what I formerly ate and loved (french fries, Burger King Whoppers and the BK Veggie, White Castle hamburgers) for what they are, i.e. nutrient deficient substitutes for God's whole foods. They are a part of Satan's plan to sabotage the Christian's right to enjoy living a God-glorifying life through good health.

CHAPTER 4

Bad Food. . . An Oxymoron

INTRODUCTION

Webster defines "food" as: "any substance taken into and assimilated by a plant or an animal to keep it alive and enable it to grow and repair tissue; nourishment; nutriment." This same dictionary defines "oxymoron" as: "figures of speech in which opposite or contradictory ideas or terms are combined."

There is no such thing as *bad* food. If we abide strictly by Webster's definition of food, it can *only* be good. If what we assimilate promotes obesity which itself can lead to heart disease, high blood pressure, sleep apnea, cancer, asthma, diabetes, and many other serious health issues, it cannot be said to promote growth and tissue repair. And it cannot be said to provide nourishment. It, therefore, by definition cannot be classified as 'food.' *Bad* food is an oxymoron. 'Food' by its very definition can only be good. Therefore if what is assimilated by the human body does what God intended it to do, then it is food. If what is assimilated by the body doesn't do what God intended it to do, it is garbage.

God says that *every herb bearing seed* and *every tree in the which is the fruit of a tree yielding seed* shall be food for man (Genesis

1:29). God's definition of food did not include anything that would promote sickness and death. Remember, after God made everything, He declared it to be *good*. Man may have altered and expanded the meaning of food to include and contain anything which we can place into our mouths despite its long-term consequences, but I'll stick to God's definition, thank you.

Paul Stitt, a former food scientist who worked for the Quaker Oats Company, got so fed up with how they and other food companies carried on their processing, that he left the food industry altogether and exposed their practices. He wrote a book about their *dirty* little secrets called *Beating the Food Giants*. Here are his thoughts concerning how "food" should be defined.

> . . . Many people distinguish between natural and 'regular'—meaning processed—foods. I couldn't agree less with that distinction. Food is not everything that fits into the mouth. In fact, the food in your supermarket basket should have to meet a very simple and very high standard. *It must nourish the human body.* In chemical analysis it must be shown to contain significant amounts of vitamins, minerals, fiber, protein, essential fatty acids and all the other growth factors which are so vital to life. . . [24]

Paul Stitt has also said that, "God never intended people to eat fake food."

Since today's fast and processed so-called food doesn't provide nearly the same benefit to man that God's original creation does, it is not food and should be avoided. I know what you're thinking. This guy is a nut, an alarmist. I probably would have thought the same thing a few months ago. But now I see the light, and my overall health, well-being, and energy is indisputable proof.

I received an email a while back which illustrates through humor American society with its ever increasing waistlines and obesity rates. When you have finished reading it, laugh heartily because it is funny. After you have finished laughing, join me in rolling up our sleeves and doing something about it. Remember,

God created you to be *healthy* and *prosperous* so that you can worship Him as He truly deserves to be worshiped.

In the beginning, God created the Heavens and the Earth and populated the Earth with broccoli, cauliflower and spinach, green and yellow and red vegetables of all kinds, so Man and Woman would live long and healthy lives. Then using God's great gifts, Satan created Ben and Jerry's Ice Cream and Krispy Creme Donuts. And Satan said, "You want chocolate with that?" And Man said, "Yes!" And Woman said, "and as long as you're at it, add some sprinkles." And they gained 10 pounds. And Satan smiled.

And God created the healthful yogurt that Woman might keep the figure that Man found so fair. And Satan brought forth white flour from the wheat, and sugar from the cane and combined them. And Woman went from size 6 to size 14.

So God said, "Try my fresh green salad." And Satan presented Thousand Island Dressing, buttery croutons and garlic toast on the side. And Man and Woman unfastened their belts following the repast.

God then said, "I have sent you heart healthy vegetables and olive oil in which to cook them." And Satan brought forth deep fried fish and chicken-fried steak so big it needed its own platter. And Man gained more weight and his cholesterol went through the roof.

God then brought forth running shoes so that His children might lose those extra pounds. And Satan gave cable TV with a remote control so Man would not have to toil changing the channels. And Man and Woman laughed and cried before the flickering blue light and gained pounds.

Then God brought forth the potato, naturally low in fat and brimming with nutrition. And Satan peeled off the healthful skin and sliced the starchy center into chips and deep-fried them. And Man gained pounds.

God then gave lean beef so that Man might consume fewer calories and still satisfy his appetite. And Satan created McDonald's and its 99-cent double-cheese-burger. Then said, "You want fries with that?" And Man replied, "Yes! And super size them!" And Satan said, "It is good." And man went into cardiac arrest.

God sighed and created quadruple bypass surgery. Then Satan created HMOs. Thought for the day:

There is more money being spent on breast implants and Viagra today than on Alzheimer's research. This means that by 2040, there should be a large elderly population with perky boobs and huge erections and absolutely no recollection of what to do with them (Author unknown).

It is a mistake to underestimate the devil. Personally I would rather *over*estimate my enemy than to *under*estimate him. "Now the serpent was *more subtil* than any beast of the field which the Lord God had made. . . "(Genesis 3:1a). One of the schemes with which Satan successfully deceives God's people is by implanting the thought, *my body is not as important as my spiritual life.* Look around you. The way we abuse our bodies through seemingly uncontrollable eating and lack of exercise is shameful.

FOOD IN THE GOOD OLD DAYS

I won't go so far as to say that food in the days when I was grow-ing up wasn't processed—some of it was. But since those days the processing has increased to the point that it cannot be categorized as 'food' anymore. The food industry has employed technology to 'improve' what we eat. They have discovered new and better methods of mass production, longer storage, and better taste and appearance, all at the expense of what is most important—growth, nourishment, health, and repair.

What has changed significantly is where we eat. *Not once*—let me repeat that to make sure you don't miss what I am about to say—*not once* did we go out to eat when I was growing up. I know what you're thinking. That was cruel and unusual punishment. To the contrary, it was a blessing. First of all, back in those days there was nowhere near the number of restaurants that we have today. And those that existed were limited in variety. ". . . In 1960, eating out was a luxury. . . there were very few choices. . . "[25] There was no choice of Chinese, Mexican, Thai, Greek, and other ethnic restaurants which are familiar today. There was maybe a choice between French meals and cafeteria food.

Second of all, my father didn't have the money to take a family out to eat which grew by one child a year until it reached ten. No one was doing it back in those early days. Not on a regular basis anyway. Eating out frequently is a rather recent development.

We ate good, nutritious, home cooked meals. By good, nutritious, and home cooked I don't mean that my mother ripped open a prepackaged meal, toss it into the microwave and call it dinner (TV dinners entered America's homes in 1954). Even if microwave ovens existed back then, my father would not have stood for that. No. My mother cooked real food, not this synthetic stuff that masquerades as food today. We had real macaroni with real cheese. On Sunday mornings she made honest to goodness *real* biscuits. What's a *real* biscuit you ask? It's a biscuit made from the basic ingredients of flour, eggs, and whatever other things she used, and mixed in a bowl. Oh, by the way, the mixer was her hands, and maybe a spoon.

When breakfast or dinner was ready, we all sat down together at the kitchen table. Everybody was there. If the meal was dinner, and we children were outside playing, my mother would call us all in to eat. If we were inside and watching television, the set would be turned off. My father would bless the food and we ate.

There was no picking and choosing from our dinner plates either. We had to eat everything on them. How many times did we hear about the children in Africa who were starving while we had so much to eat that we could throw some away? When we finished eating we had to ask our father if we could be excused from the table.

In traveling down memory lane, I am attempting to share God-glorifying family life back then. This has been abused by today's 'enlightened' society. As a consequence, family life has suffered and total health has suffered. What a trade-off! I'll take "old-school" anytime.

The amount of processed food in the supermarkets back then was nowhere near the amount we have nowadays. I remember as a youngster that we took turns accompanying our mother to the A&P supermarket on Monticello Avenue in Jersey City, New Jersey. Back then they weren't as large as they are today. I guess they had to increase the physical size in order to house the huge increase in processed (manufactured) food. Figure this one out. In just about every supermarket you'll find a small section dedicated to health foods. This is usually a gathering of organically grown foods and cereals. What does the other 95% of the supermarket contain? Unhealthy food?

Manufactured foods carried by the fast food chains, supermarkets, convenience stores, and vending machines come out of food manufacturers' chemistry labs. Remember when you took chemistry in high school or college? You performed various experiments to achieve certain results. These experiments involved mixing chemicals together. Food manufacturers do the same thing in their chemistry labs. ". . .Research on gelatin and natural broths came to an end in the 1950s when food companies discovered how to induce maillard reactions and produce meat-like flavors in the laboratory. . . "[26] The food manufacturers' purpose is to find the precise chemical additives and mixtures to make their products more appealing and tasty to the consumer. But that's not all. Their goal is also to make the product addictive, and the consumer fatter and hungrier! Who said "ignorance is bliss?"

The Center for Disease Control (CDC) in Atlanta, Georgia reported that although the number of overweight and obese women remained the same between 2000 and 2004, the same cannot be said about children and adult men. Women are not in the clear though. Their overweight and obese numbers are still very high. Overweight children increased from 14% to 17% while overweight to obese adult men increased from 27.5% to 31%. The CDC doesn't have an obese category for children. A staggering 7 out of 10 adults are overweight or obese in America!

SECRETS THE FOOD INDUSTRY WOULD RATHER KEEP SECRET

> "...In a General Foods Company report issued in 1947, chemists predicted that almost all natural flavors would soon be chemically synthesized..."[27]

Who Can You Trust? Not the food industry. Regardless of its shortcomings and bad apples, the medical establishment is far more interested in your health than the U.S. food industry is... Going to a supermarket and having to sift through a bunch of prepackaged overly processed junk...[28]

> ...Professor Kelly Brownell is head of the Rudd Center for Food Policy and Obesity at Yale, a body trying to stimulate government to change America's "toxic environment." He says the problem is the "huge amount of money to be made from a fatter population. "There are some in the Senate and House who are working hard," he told the BBC, 'but they are outnumbered by all those in the thrall of the food industry lobby.[29]

The food industry, like any other industry or company publicly traded on the New York Stock Exchange, is in business to make a profit. They are responsible to their shareholders, not to us, the consumers. "...With few exceptions, food companies are far more concerned with getting you to buy their products than they are with the nutritional value of those products. . ."[30]

A study conducted by the Quaker Oats Company in 1942 illustrates the type of callous attitude which still exists at top management in food companies. Four groups of rats were given four different diets. One group received a diet of plain whole wheat, water and synthetic vitamins and minerals. Another group received puffed wheat cereal, water, and the same synthetic vitamins and minerals the first group received. The third group was fed water and white sugar and the last group received water and the vitamins and minerals of the first and second group.

The first group of rats lived a year on their diet (whole wheat, water and synthetic vitamins and minerals). The second group lived about two weeks. The third group of rats who received water and white sugar survived for about a month. The fourth and last group lived for two months. But notice the second group, the group which was fed Quaker Oats product, puffed wheat, lived the least amount of time of all!

Paul Stitt who was formerly a food scientist at the Quaker Oats Company came across the puffed wheat rat study while doing research at the firm's library. Shocked, he showed the report to a Dr. Clark who presented it to the president of Quaker Oats, Robert D. Stuart, III. The president's reply was, "I know people should throw it on brides and grooms at weddings, but if they insist on sticking it in their mouths, can I help it? Besides, we made 9 million dollars on the stuff last year".[31]

Quaker Oats, and presumably other food companies, engage in a practice call *product differentiation*. This is a cost cutting measure and it involves making the product by a cheaper method. Although it costs less for the food companies to produce, they charge the consumer more. Also these products are even less nutritious than the original product was. Employees at Quaker Oats had to participate in taste tests during the day to see if there was any taste difference between the original product and the 'new and improved' version.

Food manufacturers use a machine called an extruder to make various shaped cereals. This process has been found to destroy the nutrient content of the cereal. Unfortunately all cereals which come in boxes, even the organic cereals sold in health food stores, are made by this process. Uh oh! I didn't know about that. I eat plenty of organic cereal. It's just that the organic cereals that I eat are not made by the publicly traded giants like Quaker Oats or Kellogg or General Mills.

James Hightower says in his book *Eat Your Heart Out: Food Profiteering in America* that these food companies are not setting out to make "bad" food, they are just not trying to make "good" food (pg. 74). As I mentioned earlier, these companies' overriding concern is profit. Processed food (food altered in a chemistry lab) is a lot more profitable than natural food. Not only is the shelf life extended indefinitely, but chemicals are added to trigger hunger and addictiveness. This leads to consumers buying more and more on a continuous basis. They do not realize that they are pumping their bodies full of poisons.

Food producers routinely put sugar in their products. It is a well known fact, especially to food manufacturers, that sugar is one of the most highly addictive substances that exist. The level at which it is addictive may vary between people, but not by much. You may find this hard to believe, but tobacco, yes the tobacco from which cigarettes are made, is cured in sugar! As a matter of fact, the tobacco companies are the largest consumers of sugar.

I can personally testify to the fact that sugar does indeed stimulate the appetite. I can eat a large bowl of organic cereal without a problem whatsoever. It's the sugar content even though the sugar is natural (such as naturally milled organic sugar, or honey). Fortunately all of the cereal I eat also contains natural, organic ingredients. Imagine all the sugar in the many different junk food cereals made by Quaker Oats, Kellogg, and General Mills. They contain tons of it and little if anything else of nutritional value. Americans consume a whopping 120 pounds of sugar per year!

It's in the food manufacturers' best interests to add sugar, lots of sugar, to their products. You see, sugar is one of the substances which cause you to overeat. There are two other substances which are added in great quantities to get you to overeat—fat and salt.

And getting you to overeat is their objective. That obviously means you must buy more of their products.

Refined sugar should be avoided, or at least minimized. It comes with a variety of names: corn syrup, high fructose corn syrup, evaporated cane juice, cane sugar, beet sugar, glucose, sucrose (refined white sugar), maltose, maltodextrin, dextrose, sorbitol, fructose, corn sugar, fruit juice concentrate, barley, malt, caramel, carob syrup to name some of the well known. These sugars are highly refined and devoid of any food value at all.

> . . . Sugar is a food processor's fantasy: it's cheap, it adds bulk and texture, and it makes consumers prefer their product over a less-sweet alternative. So now consumers get sugar everywhere, from simple carbohydrates (so called white food) to pure granulated sugar, and in other forms like dextrose, fruit juice concentrate, maltodextrin, and high-fructose corn syrup. These empty calories take the place of real nutrients. . . [32]

By law food manufacturers are not required to list all product ingredients on the label. This is loophole which the FDA (Food and Drug Administration) allows. Many of the chemicals which are listed on the labels are bad enough. Imagine the ones you don't know about. And remember, all these ingredients which are hard to pronounce are concocted in a laboratory. God did not design the human body to ingest this poison. No wonder we have all the illnesses that we do. Remember that ice cream commercial a few years back? I think it was Breyers. Johnny couldn't read the list of chemical ingredients on a rival company's ice cream label. But he had no problem reading the Breyers' list of natural ingredients. Who has trouble reading 'sugar,' 'milk'? A good rule of thumb to follow is that if you can't pronounce the ingredients, you shouldn't be eating the product.

If an ingredient, or more appropriately, a chemical, is less than 3%, the FDA does not require it to be listed on a product label. They conjecture that something in such a small quantity cannot possibly be harmful. Did you know that the bread you eat can contain oxides of nitrogen, chlorine, nitrosyl chloride, chlorine dioxide, benzoyl peroxide, acetone peroxide, and azodicarbonamide? I can guarantee you that these chemicals were not in the Garden of Eden. In Chapter 1 I mentioned that chlorine is a poison. Just because it comprises less than 3% doesn't mean that magically it is no longer a poison, and is therefore harmless. Has any study been conducted to find out the cumulative effects of these chemicals? Can anyone tell me what the effect 10 years or 20 years down the road will be? And if these chemicals are so harmless why all the secrecy? Why not list them? Hmmmmm!

Whole foods, the kinds created by God, are the kinds of food we should be eating as much as possible. These foods should be minimally processed (limited to cooking only). They certainly shouldn't be tampered with by food companies because that means they are attempting to do something with it that God did not intend. And, what's even worse, the food companies are not motivated by the consumer's health or welfare. Their motivation is one of the most selfish that man can ever allow to drive him—profit.

A personal example of the dangers of chemical additives and manufacturing processes will illustrate the danger. Up until the early part of 2006 I would mix my protein and meal replacement powders in milk. I then read the following: "milk and milk by-products are leading contributors to the $1.5 trillion sickness industry—milk causes allergies, gas, constipation, obesity, cancer, heart disease, infectious diseases, and osteoporosis"[33]

I was constantly experiencing gas and bloating during the course of a day. I had no idea what was causing it. At first I suspected the broccoli that I was eating. But I still had gas and bloating when I eliminated the broccoli from my diet. I stopped mixing my shakes in cow's milk and substituted soy milk instead. No more gas and bloating. What was it about the milk that caused my problem, and the other health problems mentioned in the book *The Wellness Revolution*?

A food biotechnology company by the name of the Monsanto Company produces a hormone known as RBGH (Recombinant Bovine Growth Hormone) which increases milk production of cows by 10% to 15%. BGH is a genetically engineered copy of the hormone which occurs naturally in cows. This hormone was approved by the FDA in 1993 and sold the next year to farmers under the name of Posilac. This hormone is banned in Canada and in Europe.

Bovine Growth Hormone is boycotted by the overwhelming majority of farmers. However the FDA, the EPA (Environmental Protection Agency), and the Department of Agriculture continue to license the hormone. This hormone has been identified as causing udder infections, reproductive and digestive problems, sores and lacerations, and other medical anomalies in cows. BGH has been linked to cancer, diabetes, and hypertension in human beings.

Studies have also shown that pasteurization changes or destroys proteins, vitamins, minerals, and enzymes in milk. This results in a number of negative health issues. Cultures have drunk raw, unpasteurized milk for centuries before Louis Pasteur discovered the process named after him. These cultures, and Americans before pasteurization, thrived on this healthy raw milk.

The real issue with the pasteurization of milk is economic, or, to get to the heart of the matter, it is a matter of profit. There's that *P* word again. Pasteurization increases the shelf life of milk. Milk straight from the cow—*un*pasteurized milk is a healthy, very nutritious food. Raw milk is unadulterated milk that God has created. I guess He knew what He was doing after all!

It seems that every day a new study comes out which points to another cause to an existing disease. The statistics about prostate cancer are alarming:

1. every 15 minutes a man dies from prostate cancer
2. every 3 minutes a case of prostate cancer is diagnosed
3. 90 percent of American men will experience some prostate deterioration by the age of 60.

There have been 16 studies which conclusively connect prostate cancer to dairy products. Pasteurized milk and cheese are loaded with pesticides, herbicides, fungicides, antibiotics, hormones and industrial toxins which attack the prostate. A Harvard study showed that only 2 ½ servings of dairy products are enough to increase the risk of contracting prostate cancer by more than 30 percent!

Complex carbohydrates which are found in whole grains such as wheat, barley and the fibrous carbohydrates contained in fruits and vegetables are not only very healthful, but they fill you up also. The food manufacturers don't want the consumer to get filled up on natural food. He wouldn't eat nearly as much of their processed food as he now does. So what do the food giants do? They refine their products by removing the complex carbohydrates and substituting artificial sweeteners and fats.

The practices of the food companies are not against the law. Neither are their practices ethical. But the Federal Drug Administration and other government agencies do not enforce ethical practices. You see, ethics interfere with achieving enormous profits at the consumers' expense. Truth be told, the FDA and other agencies are not working on our behalf. They are instead ensuring that giant food corporations make the profits that will please their shareholders and Wall Street.

As Satan deceived Eve in the garden, he has deceived us. We have been duped into thinking that God's provisions have somehow become less than satisfactory. And this is after centuries of successfully providing health and vitality. We have swallowed the convincing lies perpetrated by doctors, scientists, and the giant food manufacturers that their processes and chemical additives are now necessary. Not only have we allowed Satan to destroy our health, we have allowed him to use this issue to decimate the family as well.

Much of what I have written has come from 'insider' information. Just as we had no idea of the deceptions and unscrupulous practices of the tobacco industry until Dr. Jeffrey Wigand exposed them, so it is with the food companies. Paul Stitt has exposed the inside practices of the food industry. Thank God for these men. It took courage to make this information public. Now that it is out in the open, we can take steps to get our physical bodies closer to what God our Creator intended for them to be.

Foods to Avoid

I guess by now you're wondering if there is anything left to eat. Yes there is. Although you may think so, I am not attempting to deprive you of the pleasure of eating. I enjoy eating myself. But anything can become a god to you. If food *controls* you, then that is your god. Our God is a jealous God and He says that we are not to have any other gods besides Him (Exodus 20:3)! You just have to make better food choices and learn to read food product labels. Fast food franchises such as McDonald's, Burger King, White Castle and all the others should be avoided. These places do not sell food. They sell great tasting items which have been so processed and chemically altered that they make you gain a lot of unhealthy weight (fat) and create life threatening health issues.

I used to eat at these places. But since I have read and studied the motives, ingredients, methods of preparation, and the accompanying health dangers, I have since stopped. If you are patronizing these fast food franchises on a regular basis, I would recommend gradually cutting back. They are certainly no substitute for healthy, home-prepared meals. If you absolutely have to eat fast food, I would not recommend going more than once a month.

The body has to be retrained. I am speaking to you from experience. My body had come to crave the large amounts of salt, fat, and sugar I was feeding it when I patronized fast food restaurants. I retrained my body by gradually depriving it of the unnecessary amounts of fats, sugars, and salt I was putting into it. I am now at the point where the skin on chicken and turkey (fat) is repulsive to me. I also don't need to add additional salt to my meals (what is already present is more than enough).

Below is a list of things that are to be avoided *at all costs*. Not only will they prevent one from living a God-glorifying life, but they will contribute to chronic health problems, and possibly death. You won't find anything in this list that is found naturally in nature. That means they are synthetic and toxic to the body. They were created in chemical laboratories by food companies who only care about the *almighty buck*!

TRANS FATS

God has created the water and food that man needs to live on, but unfortunately additives and processes have turned healthy, life sustaining substances into deadly poisons. Water is absolutely essential for human, animal, and plant life. But we have found that by adding fluoride and chlorine to it, it becomes toxic. Raw cow's milk is both nutritious and healthy. But the process of homogenization and pasteurization destroys its health benefits.

The process of hydrogenation which yields trans fatty acids was invented by the German scientist Wilhelm Normann in 1902. During the early to mid '80s there was a public outcry against saturated fats in fast food products. The Center for Science in the Public Interest (CSPI) officially voiced opposition to the use of saturated fats. In response, the fast food industry replaced saturated fats with trans fats. When studies showed that trans fats were worse then saturated fats, CSPI campaigned against them in 1992.

Natural vegetable oil becomes extremely dangerous when man tampers with it. *Trans fatty acids should be avoided at all costs.* Trans fatty acids, also known as trans fat, are created by injecting hydrogen gas into a vat of vegetable oil. The objective is to get the contents to become partially solid margarine or shortening. Crisco Oil and margarine are trans fats. Food manufacturers like these products because they have a much longer shelf life than butter and they are cheaper to make. By the way, contrary to what has been advertised by the food companies, butter is better for you than margarine. On a product's ingredient label, trans fat is listed as *partially hydrogenated vegetable oil*, or *hydrogenated vegetable oil*, or *shortening*. Ingredients are listed in the order of the amount present in the product from greater to lesser.

Besides shortening and margarine, partially hydrogenated vegetable oils are found in fried foods such as french fries and chicken. Baked goods such as donuts, cookies and crackers also contain this oil. Some breakfast cereals and waffles as well as candy, snack foods, salad dressings, and other processed foods contain trans fats. Trans fats increase the levels of bad cholesterol and decrease the levels of good cholesterol. They clog the arteries and can lead to heart disease which is the nation's number one killer. ". . . Many, many diseases have been associated with the consumption of these trans fatty acids—heart disease, cancer, and degeneration of joints and tendons (that is why we have so many hip replacements today). . ."[34]

Again, *all* products with trans fats should be avoided!

Trans fats are in a great majority of the processed food which is purchased in the supermarket, food marts, convenience stores, and vending machines. And they are found in the fried products at the fast food restaurants. *All processed food should be avoided.* Food should be eaten in the way we find it in nature. An alternative is to patronize a health food store. There you can purchase snacks made with organic ingredients and no chemical preservatives. These health food stores have cookies and other pastries to satisfy that 'sweet' tooth along with natural potato chips with organic sea salt. And, don't forget, organic fruit has God's sweetener already in it. You can eat as much as you like and not have to worry about going into cardiac arrest. I prefer the fruit to the juice. The process of pasteurization can destroy some vitamins and minerals. And with the fruit, you're also getting the fiber.

> "Order french fries or hot wings at a McDonald's or a KFC in the United States and you're more likely to get a super-size helping of artery-clogging trans fats than you would at their restaurants in some other countries. . ."[35]

Steen Stender, one of the researchers of the above study, is a cardiologist at Gentofte University Hospital in Hellerup, Denmark. He remarked that he was astonished to see such a wide variation of trans fat content. Commenting further, Stender said ". . . per gram, it is more harmful than any other kind of fat. . . it's a metabolic poison. . ."[36]

The United States was one of the countries which have the highest amounts of trans fat. Partially hydrogenated vegetable oils don't go bad and it can be used over and over again at a considerable cost savings. Denmark was the only country in the test where laws prohibit partially hydrogenated vegetable oil from being used.

A recent study has revealed that as bad as trans fat is, it is even more deadly than previously thought. A study conducted by scientific researchers at Wake Forest University on velvet monkeys found that trans fats not only made the monkeys fatter by adding new fat, but that the trans fats also redistributed fat from other areas of the body to the stomach. The monkeys were fed a typical western diet consisting of 35 percent fat. Their diet was calorie controlled and they should not have gained any weight at all (on paper). Trans fat caused the monkeys to increase their weight by 7.2 percent compared to the 1.8 percent increase in the monkeys who were given unsaturated fats. Fat concentrated in the abdominal region increases the risk for diabetes and heart disease.

HIGH FRUCTOSE CORN SYRUP

> ... To shed fat, you must wean yourself off foods that contain an additive called high-fructose corn syrup (HFCS)... Not only does fructose turn preferentially into fat, it also shuts down the mechanisms your body has for preventing fat accumulation... [37]

> When you and I were in grade school, there might have been one heavy kid in our class. But now there might be only one kid who's not overweight. Why? A new study just concluded that 9 out of 10 adult men (and 7 in 10 women) will become overweight before they die. Even if you're fit and trim now, watch out—you're doomed to balloon. Why?[38]

Fructose is fruit sugar found naturally in fruits and vegetables. The amount of this natural, God created sugar is small but it is in addition to the fiber and vitamins. The fiber in the fruit and vegetable slows down the metabolism of the fructose. But leave it to man to pervert what God has made to benefit the body in order to give man a heightened taste experience. High Fructose Corn Syrup (HFCS) is made by treating a large quantity of glucose with an enzyme that changes part of the glucose into a much sweeter fructose. HFCS is cheaper than cane sugar and it is inexpensively produced. Without the fiber and other natural nutrients of fruit and vegetables, HFCS is rapidly absorbed into the bloodstream.

Food manufacturers began using HFCS in the 1970s. The per capita use of HFCS in 1970 was ½ pound. By 1997 the average American use of HFCS was an astounding 97 grams per day! This equates to 78 pounds per year! Today its use has increased tremendously, contributing to this country's rising obesity epidemic. The product which contains the greatest number of grams of HFCS is soft drinks. It is also found in candy, ice cream, frozen yogurt, Popsicles, fruit bars, ketchup, pasta sauce, soups, and hamburger buns (this list is by no means exhaustive!)

When food manufacturers first began using HFCS they didn't realize its negative impact on the body. That was then. But since then food manufacturers have discovered that HFCS not only make consumers fat, but it also increases their hunger tremendously. That's bad for the consumer but good for the food manufacturers. The hungrier the consumer, the more food they will buy. The more food that is purchased the greater the manufacturers' profit. Cha-ching! They could care less about the rising obesity and medical crisis.

Soda contains the greatest amount of HFCS while carrying no nutritive value at all. It is total garbage. If man made it, you should not feed it to your body. Try drinking more water. You can also drink 100% fruit juice. Avoid fruit *drinks* because they contain HFCS also. Many people substitute diet sodas for regular soda thinking that they are drinking fewer calories. However a recent study has found that diet sodas contributed more to the rising obesity epidemic than regular soda!

High Fructose Corn Syrup is a product of the chemistry lab. It is much sweeter than regular table sugar. As a matter of fact, it is far better to buy unsweetened cereal or yogurt, and sweeten it yourself with table sugar. You can be sure that you will add less than is present in commercially prepared foods. And although table sugar has been processed, it is less dangerous and additive than the artificial sweeteners so widely used today.

MONOSODIUM GLUTAMATE (MSG)

Monosodium glutamate is a compound known as an *exitotoxin*. Exitotoxins are proteins which make brain cells fire their impulses rapidly when they make contact with it. The cells become so hyper-excited that they continue to fire until the cell is exhausted, and subsequently die. Naturally this is an abnormal situation and can only happen when man tampers with God's perfect food and water supply.

> Why is free glutamic acid added in vast amounts to processed foods? Our large profit-driven food companies have found that manufactured free glutamic acid, in the form of monosodium glutamate (MSG), hydrolyzed vegetable proteins, etc., etc., when added to our processed foods, masks off flavors and makes the blandest and cheapest foods taste wonderful. . . [39]

What began thousands of years ago in Japan as an all-natural flavor enhancer found in kombu, an edible kelp, and other natural sources such as seaweed, has become a source of enormous profits for the food industry. In 1908 a Japanese scientist isolated the active ingredient in kombu which was responsible for the exciting flavor of the foods it was added to. It was glutamic acid. This ingredient was discovered by the Americans during World War II after eating Japanese food rations. After the war, monosodium glutamate was given to the food industry. Since then, its use has exploded and even now shows no signs of slowing down.

Monosodium glutamate isn't just sensed by the taste buds in our tongues, it also triggers and excites the neurons in the brain. Free glutamic acid is able to reach the brain where it can injure and kill the neurons. A quarter of the American people are susceptible to glutamic acid causing a wide range of negative reactions. This acid doesn't cause a problem in anyone when it is a part of whole, natural, God created unprocessed food. It becomes a problem when man separates it through a chemical process in a laboratory. Monosodium glutamate which is a part of processed food is hidden in ingredients going by many different and confusing names.

> ... Monosodium glutamate and other forms of free glutamic acid can be manufactured cheaply and sometimes it is even just a by-product of other food processes. For example, the brewer's yeast from the brewing industry contains free glutamic acid. Since free glutamic acid is cheap and since its neurotoxic nerve stimulation enhances so wonderfully the flavor of basically bland and tasteless foods, such as many low-fat and vegetarian foods, manufacturers are eager to go on using it and do not want the public to realize any of the problems. . . "[40]

> ... The fast food industry could not exist without MSG and artificial meat flavors to make secret sauces and spice mixes that beguile the consumer into eating bland and tasteless food. The sauces in processed food are basically MSG, water, some thickener and emulsifier and some caramel coloring. Your tongue is tricked into thinking that it is getting something nutritious when it is getting nothing at all except some very toxic substances. . . [41]

Monosodium glutamate is ubiquitous. The taste that it gives processed food is addictive. MSG is also a major contributor to the obesity epidemic. It makes manufactured food taste so good that we can't get enough of it. Remember the television commercial about Lay's potato chips (FritoLay Corp), 'bet you can't eat just one?' Not only is that statement true of potato chips, but all the other manufactured products that we purchase at fast food restaurants (including pizza parlors) and at the supermarket.

Not only is MSG responsible toward contributing to the skyrocketing obesity health crisis, but also the following health issues: migraine headaches, sleeping disorders, IBS (Irritable Bowel Syndrome), asthma, diabetes, Alzheimer's disease, Lou Gehrig's disease, ADD (Attention Deficit Disorder), seizures and strokes. And the list includes more! Very, very few doctors, dieticians, or the general public are aware of these toxic dangers which MSG can produce.

No one knows exactly how much MSG we consume. It is not all explicitly put on food labels. But the amount is *too much*! There are many ingredients (or shall I call them what they really are, chemicals?) that the FDA allows food manufacturers not to list on its labels. Even labels which say 'No MSG' or 'No MSG Added' are deceptive. MSG can be produced during food processing. So technically, none is added. Even the label 'all natural' is deceptive because the FDA considers monosodium glutamate 'natural.'

The following *ALWAYS contain* MSG:

> *glutamate*
> *monosodium glutamate*
> *monopotassium glutamate*
> *glutamic acid*
> *calcium caseinate*
> *gelatin*
> *textured protein*
> *hydrolyzed protein* (any protein that is hydrolyzed)
> *yeast extract*
> *yeast food*
> *autolyzed yeast*
> *yeast nutrient*

The following list often contains MSG, or it is created during processing:

> *natural flavors*
> *natural pork flavoring*

Bouillon
natural beef flavoring
stock natural chicken flavoring
broth
malt flavoring
barley malt
malt extract
seasonings
carrageenan
soy sauce
soy sauce extract
soy protein
soy protein concentrate
soy protein isolate
pectin
maltodextrin
whey protein
whey protein isolate
whey protein concentrate
protease
protease enzymes
enzymes
anything *ultra-pasteurized*
anything *fermented*

Some of my protein supplements contained MSG, or MSG was created during processing. I have replaced these products. I have eliminated all other sources that I am aware of from my diet as well. That means I have reduced the total amount of MSG that I ingest to a bare minimum. I buy all organic foods (meats, veggies, fruits, cereals, soy milk) and don't patronize fast food restaurants anymore. I do my food shopping exclusively at Whole Foods. I don't go out to eat that often, but when I do, I make the most intelligent choices I can.

Scientists began noticing problems with MSG in 1957. Experimenting on mice, they discovered that these mice became blind and obese as a direct result of being fed MSG. In 1969 lesions produced by MSG were found in the brain. MSG has been found to adversely affect the brain causing problems ranging from headaches to permanent brain damage. "... We have a huge increase in Alzheimer's, brain cancer, seizures, multiple sclerosis and diseases of the nervous system and one of the chief reasons is these flavorings in our food. MSG is also associated with violent behavior..."[42]

Beginning in the late 1950s, MSG was added in large amounts to baby food. Read a food label of a baby food product. If one of the ingredients is *hydrolyzed protein*, it is MSG disguised under another name. As it stands, about 95% of processed food contain MSG.

SOY

> Vegetarians and health enthusiasts have known for years that foods rich in soy protein offer a good alternative to meat, poultry, and other animal-based products. As consumers have pursued healthier lifestyles in recent years, consumption of soy foods has raised steadily, bolstered by scientific studies showing health benefits from these products. Last October, the Food and Drug Administration gave food manufacturers permission to put labels on products high in soy protein indicating that these foods may help lower heart disease risk... [43]

Despite this glowing testimonial by the FDA (Food and Drug Administration), continuing research has found that all may not be well in the world of soy. It may not be the "superfood" that many of its proponents thought it was. As of last year, my chief source of protein powder has been soy isolate. I have a protein drink anywhere from 2 to 3 times a day. This form of soy is particularly problematic. It is on the list of foods which may contain MSG or MSG is created during processing (Refer to Monosodium Glutamate above). To add to the problem, 99 percent of soy is genetically modified.

Listed is a summary of what recent and continuing research has found out about soy:

1. *Phytates* these are phosphorous compounds found primarily in cereal grains, legumes, and nuts (of course soy is included). Phytates bind with the minerals calcium, magnesium, copper, zinc, and iron and disrupts the body's absorption of them. Diets high in phytates have been found to interfere with a child's normal growth. There are other camps which see phytates' role as removing excess minerals from the body and bolstering the immune system.

2. *Phytoestrogens (isoflavones)* phytoestrogens have the ability to copy the effects of estrogen, the female hormone. Infants should not be given soy based formulas at all. Although the FDA regulates products which contain estrogen, they are silent about soy. Phytoestrogens could possibly cause infertility in women and lead to breast cancer. Two senior toxicologists who are with the FDA have stated that the public is at risk from soy isoflavones in soy protein isolate. Phytoestrogens genistein and daidzein are especially problematic.

3. *Enzyme inhibitors* interfere with the digestion of protein and may cause pancreatic disorders.

4. *Haemaggluttin* causes red blood cells to bind together and hinder oxygen take-up.

The potential problems which have been covered do not apply to fermented soy products such as natto, soybean sprouts, tempeh, and miso. The process of fermentation nullifies the phytates in soy. Probiotics are created during this process. These are good bacterium which assists the body in the absorption and digestibility of nutrients.

My research into soy seems to point in the direction of soy protein isolate as a major culprit. I use the Silk brand of soy milk. Silk uses whole soy beans, not the protein isolate. Neither is their beans genetically modified. Some of the problems may still exist even with the Silk process, but I am comfortable that their milk poses less of a threat than other brands, and all products using soy protein isolate. I have found a substitute for my protein powder (fermented soy protein). It seems that although everyone may be susceptible to some of the dangers of soy, women and infants seem to be especially vulnerable.

Based on what studies and research has shown, only use soy that is organically grown and has been fermented. It should not be genetically modified in any way. You can purchase organically grown and fermented soy protein powder at this site:

www.nutritiongeeks.com

ARTIFICIAL SWEETENERS

Artificial sweeteners, also known as sugar substitutes, are man-made chemical substances used in place of table sugar (sucrose). These sweeteners are many times sweeter than table sugar so that much less is needed to produce the same level of sweetness as table sugar.

Saccharine. Believe it or not but saccharine has been in existence since 1879. It is 300 times sweeter than ordinary table sugar. We are most familiar with saccharine in the form of *Sweet 'N Low.* In 1977 a Canadian study proved that saccharine caused bladder cancer in laboratory rats. Because of this study, the Federal Drug Administration required that all products containing saccharine carry the following warning: *"Use of this product may be hazardous to your health. This product contains saccharine, which has been determined to cause cancer in laboratory animals."*

Due to the conclusive nature of the Canadian study, and the fact that further studies were conducted in the United States, the FDA wanted to ban saccharine altogether. The food industry successfully fought against this ban. After all, this sweetener was in so many products, especially regular and diet sodas. It is bringing in millions of dollars in profit. It is a 'cash cow' to soda manufacturers. "... People who drank only 2 cans or more of diet soda had an increased risk..."[44]

Food manufacturers are interested in one thing, and one

thing only, money. They are driven purely by the enormous profits that they are raking in, especially with the deception of the *diet* fad movement. Their collective consciousnesses are not disturbed in the least by the fact that saccharine is a proven cancer producer. "For the love of money is the root of all evil. . . " (I Timothy 6:10a).

> . . . Pregnant mothers are especially cautioned to stay away from saccharine because even small usage of saccharine could overwhelm the developing fetus' defenses and cause damage to the developing bladder area. . . Saccharine is cheap and stable so diet food makers find it perfect for use in sodas, candies, and many other products. . . [45]

Aspartame. This artificial sweetener is an *exitotoxin*. It was discovered in 1965 and is 200 times sweeter than table sugar. It can be found in over 5,000 products all over the world including carbonated drinks and various foods.

Aspartame is formed when two amino acids and a methyl group are joined together. However, upon digestion, methanol is formed. This is a dangerous chemical and it is strictly controlled by the EPA (Environmental Protection Agency). The level of methanol that the EPA allows in aspartame is 7 times what it allows anyone else to use! You may recognize aspartame under the popular name NutraSweet. It is also sold as Equal. I don't know about you, but I see the food industry exerting a strong influence on the EPA. So what else is new? The food industry, like Big Pharma, has powerful lobbyists in Washington and millions of dollars to spend in protecting its interests.

NutraSweet has been associated with seizures and multiple sclerosis. It can also precipitate ADD (attention deficit disorder) and ADHD (attention deficit hyperactive disorder). NutraSweet changes cell function and can cause children to become violent and hyperactive. Drinking this chemical over long periods of time can cause permanent brain damage.

NutraSweet gradually became popular when the dangers of

saccharine were made public. But this artificial sweetener is just as bad. It is also addictive and contributes to obesity.

Sucralose. This sweetener is more popularly known as *Splenda*. Splenda is produced by the pharmaceutical giant, Johnson & Johnson. Contrary to advertising campaigns, sucralose is not natural like fructose (fruit sugar) or lactose (milk sugar). Instead of being produced by nature, it is produced in a chemical laboratory.

Sucralose contains chlorine atoms. Chlorine is a poison. Sucralose is 600 times sweeter than sugar. There have been no long-term studies to find out the effects of Splenda in humans.

> "... There have been no long-term human studies conducted to determine the potential health effects of Splenda on humans, including children. Until long-term human studies are conducted, no one will know for sure whether Splenda is really safe or unsafe to eat..."[46]

Splenda can be found in almost 3,500 food products. And remember, when you consume Splenda, you are consuming the deadly poison chlorine. In its tests, the FDA has found out that up to 27% of sucralose can be absorbed by the human body. Never forget, Splenda, like all the other artificial sweeteners, are made in chemical laboratories. That is why they are called *artificial*. I can guarantee you that Adam and Eve did not have, nor did they need man-made chemicals. Everything needed for physical pleasure and nutrition was provided by God. They also didn't have a weight problem. This is an abnormal condition caused by man's irresponsibility and his rampant technology.

WHITE SUGAR, WHITE FLOUR, WHITE RICE

White Table Sugar. Anytime man takes a natural substance and strips something away from it or adds to it through chemicals or other processing methods, he renders God's creation impotent and weak, and *dangerous*! Raw sugar is good and nutritious. White table sugar has undergone so much processing that all nutritional value is removed, and it has become a drug as lethal as any illegal drug could be.

Natural unprocessed sugar is brownish in color and could rightly be called a 'food.' The white table sugar that you are familiar with has been bleached with a chemical. Brown sugar is no better. It is merely white table sugar with a little molasses put back in. Americans consume so much sugar in the form of HFCS (High Fructose Corn Syrup), artificial sweeteners, and table sugar that it qualifies to be classified as *substance abuse*. A 12 ounce container of your typical soft drink can have as much as nine teaspoons of sugar in it. The average person eats 130 pounds of sugar a year!

> ... In other studies, chronic violence in prisons was remarkably reduced simply by eliminating refined sugar and starch from prison diets. Singapore in 1991 banned sugary soft drink sales from all schools and youth centers, citing the danger that sugar poses to the mental and physical health of children... [47]

Since white table sugar is deficient in nutrients, body resources have to be used in its metabolism. What am I saying? It takes nutrients to process sugar. If these nutrients are not present in the bloodstream, the body will cannibalize its own tissue to get them. It's like 'robbing Peter to pay Paul.' Vitamins and minerals are needed to metabolize or process sugar. If these are in short supply, the body will seek them from muscle tissue and bone. And the result is the *domino effect*. Robbing muscle tissue of essential vitamins and minerals leaves the body depleted of these nutrients, and hungry. And since Americans overdose on sugar, and don't get enough exercise, or don't exercise at all, the sugar is stored as fat. Do you see what's happening? Hunger and sugar cravings? The food industry couldn't be more pleased. You are now stuffed and plump like a Thanksgiving turkey, and suffering from all sorts of medical problems as a result. Your doctor now prescribes prescription drugs (other poisons) to cover the symptoms of the real problem—*too* much sugar and *too* much processed food. And the vicious cycle continues.

Instead of white sugar, use organic honey, organic fruit juice, or evaporated sugar cane juice.

White Rice. Rice is a grain. In nature it is brown in color. White rice is brown rice with its husk, bran, and germ removed. The process removes most of the fiber and nutrients. The body thus treats white rice as a simple carbohydrate. And, like sugar, it is rapidly absorbed into the bloodstream. The blood sugar shoots sky high and then comes plummeting down. Fiber, which God in His infinite wisdom provided in natural brown rice, prevents the blood sugar roller coaster ride. Needless to say, brown rice is much more nutritious than white rice.

White Flour. Like rice, wheat is a grain. It is naturally brown in color. Whole wheat is naturally high in fiber and vitamins and minerals. Eating anything but organic whole wheat is to introduce chemically processed substances into your body. You want *organic* whole wheat because you want wheat that was grown pesticide and herbicide free. You want *whole* wheat because you don't want any bleaching process used or any of its nutrients removed.

Remember earlier in this book I told you that my father made us put wheat germ on our food? Well wheat germ is the heart of the wheat kernel. It is chock full of B vitamins such as folate, thiamin, and vitamin B6; it also contains the minerals zinc, magnesium, and manganese. The brand of wheat germ that my father used was Kretschmer.

If the label doesn't say *whole* wheat (as in 100% whole wheat), than the product is a mixture of enriched white bread and whole wheat. That's no good. You want 100% whole wheat. White bread has been stripped of its fiber and nutrient content and then bleached. *Enriched* means that some of the nutrients were put back in. Duh? Why remove them in the first place? The enriching process only returns four vitamins and minerals to the flour and none of the fiber.

The bleaching process used to turn natural brown wheat flour into a pretty and glistening white but totally lifeless flour always leaves residuals behind. Some of the chemical bleaches used are oxide of nitrogen, chlorine (there's that poison again), chloride, nitrosyl, and benzoyl peroxide. And these are mixed with various salts.

Remember what I said my father told me? White bread was used as paste to hang wallpaper. Uuughh! Think of what it's doing to your insides. White refined flour is a natural insecticide. If any insect were to get into a sack of white flour, it would soon die. White flour is poison. What to do? Stop eating all processed, refined white flour products. This includes, but is not limited to white bread, hamburger and hot dog rolls, breakfast rolls, and any other baked goods which use processed flour.

You know the saying 'an educated consumer is our best customer?' Well, in the case of food processors and their engineered foods, this might not be true. If the consumer knew the truth about not only the food companies' products, but the deceptive advertising that they perpetrate to lure their victim, excuse me, I mean customer, he would be a *former* customer. It is in the food companies' best interests that the consumer remains ignorant of and uneducated to the foods he eats.

Personally speaking, I discovered the truth about the agenda of the food companies through the book *Natural Cures "They" Don't Want You To Know About*. That was the beginning of the end between me and these food companies and their unnatural and unhealthy products. I was ignorant for 53 years. John 8:32 says "And ye shall know the truth, and the truth shall make you free." Because I was ignorant of the full truth about processed foods, and totally ignorant about God receiving glory through a completely healthy and maintained body, I was in bondage. But now I have been 'made' free.

"Lest Satan should get an advantage of us; for we are
not ignorant of his devices" (II Corinthians 2:11).

The devil will use anything and everything to prevent a Christian from experiencing an abundant life in Christ. He knows that most Christians are focused on the spiritual life only. He desires to keep us in the dark concerning the total man—spirit, soul, *and* body. Satan would have you believe that concern with the physical man is nothing less than egotism—a focus on *self*. Nothing could be further from the truth. Satan would have you conveniently forget that it was God who created the body. And that reverence for God means reverence for that which God has created. I didn't say we should 'worship' the body, but we are to 'reverence' it.

God told Adam that He has given him every tree in the garden from which to eat, with the exception of one. He didn't leave it up to man to create his own menu. God designed and made nutritious and delicious food which was complete with all the nutrients which Adam needed. An adherence to God's natural and whole food meant that Adam's body would never get sick. Adam didn't have to seek after Satan's synthetic foods which do not benefit the human body that God gave him.

The devil is a counterfeiter. For the true which God has created, Satan has a counterfeit—a false. And his counterfeit is always without exception booby trapped with danger. Notice that the grass always looks greener on the other side? Satan's counterfeit food is loaded with toxins, and is designed to weaken and destroy the body. Then Satan presents his toxic (synthetic) drugs which he convincingly says you need in order to 'cure' the medical condition brought on by his counterfeit food.

The devil's plan is well thought out. It has been successful for thousands of years. It is the same plan which trapped Eve. "And when the woman saw that the tree was good for food and that it was pleasant to the eyes..." (Genesis 3:6a).' Look at that pretty white bread' Satan whispers to you. 'It's much better for you than that ugly brown bread.' Don't be fooled by the devil's lie. Look at the price Adam and Eve had to pay. A constant diet of the devil's food will lead to devastating medical problems, and then to a steady regimen of toxic prescription drugs and financial ruin. By then your body will be weak and run down, nutritionally depleted, subject to colds, the flu, and the *I don't feel like doing anything today* attitude.

When the devil has your body weak and wracked with pain, he has accomplished his goal. It is impossible to live a God-glorifying life through good health in that state. God desires for His children to be over comers and victorious in all aspects of their lives. This is easy to accomplish. I am a living witness. I am not a slave to junk food or to toxic prescription and nonprescription drugs. Neither am I victimized by cancer, hypertension, diabetes, colds, heart disease, asthma, aches and pains, sluggishness, arthritis, or any of the other dozens of ailments brought on by poor nutrition and no exercise.

You *don't* need prescription and nonprescription drugs to mask the symptoms of your *real* problem. What you need to ask yourself is: *Why do I have diabetes? Why do I have high blood pressure? Why do I have cancer? Why do I have heart disease?* These are the issues that Satan doesn't want you to focus on. If he can keep you focused on the *symptom* (asthma, hypertension, etc), rather than the *cause* (white flour, MSG, HFCS, artificial sweeteners, etc. which are poisonous to the body), then Satan can keep you addicted to prescription and nonprescription drugs, and to the toxic products which passes for food from the food companies. And ultimately this will hasten your physical demise (shorter life span) and prevent you from experiencing the abundant life which Christ has promised you.

In order to experience the abundant life in Christ physically, a change in lifestyle must be made. The disrespect and irreverence of the body which God has given you have to stop. In its place a completely new lifestyle must be adopted. This new lifestyle encompasses a return to the whole food which God has placed on earth (this means unprocessed and unrefined) and a consistent program of exercise. God has also given us doctors who believe in *alternative* cures (natural medicines made from herbs and other natural substances). They should be sought out so that the body can be weaned off the toxic and synthetic drugs made by Big Pharma.

Are there any guarantees in going back to God's way? Yes. The guarantee is given in the Word of God. And I am your living and breathing witness. Feel and be as you've never felt and been before. You'll be so healthy and energetic that you will soon forget what it feels like to be ill and *pooped out* and sluggish all the time. You'll forget what it feels like to have to take those synthetic drugs, which do nothing but harm to the body. As a matter of fact, you'll feel as though you could *run through a troop* and *leap over a wall* (Psalms 18:29) even though you're over 50, or 60, or 80.

TABLE SALT

Many of us think nothing of dumping salt on food. Since we habitually pour salt on just about everything we eat, our taste buds and our brain tell us that the food we eat is bland without it. I don't remember what sparked me to change my use of salt, but I did decades ago. I retrained my taste buds and brain. Now I don't put salt on anything. I don't need it.

Ordinary table salt is 97.5% sodium chloride. Sodium chloride is in just about all preserved, process food. The majority of the food the typical American eats is processed. This means that most people use much too much salt. Like white rice, bread, flour, and sugar, table salt is not natural. It is chemically processed. The other 2.5% of table salt is composed of moisture absorbents and iodine. The salt is dried at 1200 degrees Fahrenheit, which drastically changes its molecular structure. Since its molecular structure has been changed, the body does not recognize it. This can lead to serious health issues.

An average American uses 4,000 to 6,000 mg (milligrams) of salt daily, and some use up to 10,000 mg! Clearly these figures are not unlike overdosing on drugs. Excessive salt use causes the body to retain fluid (water). Health problems such as cellulite, rheumatism, arthritis, gout, and kidney and gall bladder stones are all attributable to excessive salt use. Aluminum hydroxide is also added to table salt to help it pour. When aluminum is ingested, it is stored in the brain. Medical science has found out that aluminum may be a contributing cause of Alzheimer's disease.

UNDERSTANDING DECEPTIVE FOOD LABELS

Food companies have advertising budgets in the millions of dollars to come up with *deceptive* food labeling. Though not obvious out and out lies, the labels and catch phrases are designed to make you think and feel a certain way. And most important of all, they are designed to make you want to purchase the product. What is the truth behind the clever phrases? The hype? Are you confused by "fat free," "reduced fat," "no fat," "low fat," "low carb," or "sugar free?" I sure was.

You are the typical the consumer who honestly wants to lose weight. You are confronted with all these phrases. What is the difference between them? Does it matter which you choose? Will you get "slim and trim" by using them?

In any discussion about fat, one fact should be made clear. Unlike man, all fats are not created equal. All fats are not bad. The fat that should be avoided altogether is trans fatty acids, or trans fat. Saturated fats (beef, pork) should be kept to a minimum. There are heart healthy fats called monounsaturated and omega 3s that should be included in abundance in the diet. Polyunsaturated fats should also be in the diet but to a lesser extent.

REDUCED FAT

The official definition of "reduced fat" is: product has at least 25% less fat than the original product. But what if the fat that is reduced to achieve the "reduced fat" designation is monounsaturated, the good fat? And if the total calories are the same, then the manufacturer has probably added more sugar and/or chemicals. Obviously this is not what you would want. My recommendation is not to play games with food manufacturers. Buy your food at a health food store, or your local organic food supermarket. But still read the label.

LOW FAT

Product contains 3 or less grams of fat per serving. Food companies often compensate for the loss of texture and taste resulting from the removal of fat by adding sugar. Hello! Slick, aren't they? But you're not going to be fooled anymore. Here's a good example. Ben & Jerry's Chocolate Fudge Brownie *Low-Fat* Frozen Yogurt contains 190 calories composed of 2.5 grams of fat and 36 grams of carbohydrates per serving. Breyers Chocolate Ice Cream has 160 total calories with 9 grams of fat and 18 grams of carbohydrates per serving. So you see, even though Ben & Jerry's is a *low fat* yogurt, it contains 30 more calories and 18 more grams of carbs than Breyers ice cream! You are better off with Breyers. I will not lie to you, I love ice cream.

FAT FREE

"Fat free" products have less than ½ gram of fat in a serving. Technically "fat free" means *no fat at all—zero—zippo*! I consider this phrase to be deceptive, don't you?

LOW CARB

There are no government regulations as to what could be considered "low carb." There are simple carbohydrates and complex carbohydrates. The simple carbs are things like sugar (table sugar, fruit sugar, honey, etc). These carbs are quickly absorbed into the bloodstream and raise blood levels. Fruits are good. Eat plenty of them. However stay away from refined or processed sugars (candies, pies, cakes, table sugar, etc). except for an occasional treat. Complex carbohydrates on the other hand are things like veggies, sweet potatoes, bran, wheat, brown rice, etc. Eat plenty of these foods as they are slowly absorbed and have a lot of fiber.

There is plenty of room for customer fraud here. One food manufacturer labeled his cookies 'low carb' simply because the serving size was listed as two cookies as compared to the regular cookies' serving size of three. Not only will food companies do just about anything to make a buck, they will insult your intelligence in the process. I don't know about you, but I hate having my intelligence insulted. I don't bother with the games these publicly traded food companies' play anymore (which is to say I don't buy any of their products). If I want cookies or cakes, I purchase them at a health food store and make sure that all of the ingredients are 100% organic. Just be sure not to overdose on portion sizes.

It's unfortunate that many people seem to think that just because a product says "low fat" or "low carb" they can eat as many as they want. What you have to remember is a calorie is a calorie. Even if a product is legitimately "low carb," eating too many will still pack on the pounds. "Low carb" is *not* a license to eat more.

> . . . So in the end the lesson learned is that we must be cautious of food labeling! Companies are very good at marketing their products around our health concerns as well as manipulating the nutrition guidelines. . . If a food seems too good to be true, it probably is!"[48]

NATURAL, ALL NATURAL, 100% NATURAL

What does the typical consumer think when he or she hears the word "natural" in relationship to a food product or a drink? Well I'm a typical consumer and I associate "natural" with "ingredients from nature" and with "health." Unfortunately the FDA (Food and Drug Administration) does not have an official, iron-clad definition of "natural." Currently it considers a product natural if it contains "nothing artificial or synthetic," and it doesn't contain anything that the consumer wouldn't normally expect to find in a product. In contrast to the FDA's ambiguous policy, the USDA (United States Department of Agriculture) defines "natural" as meat and poultry that has been minimally processed.

Let me give you an example of what is being accepted by the FDA as "natural." Ben & Jerry's all natural ice cream contains hydrogenated oil, corn syrup, alkalized cocoa powder, and artificial flavors. Big joke isn't it? Now contrast Ben & Jerry's "all natural" ice cream with Breyers all natural ice cream. If you read Breyers' list of ingredients (Vanilla Swiss Almond) you will find: cream, sugar, natural flavor, natural tara gum, butter oil and other natural ingredients. Breyers is the better choice. Now I am not advocating that ice cream be added to your diet. Natural or not, it is still fattening. Are consumers going to have to hire lawyers to help them understand 'slick' advertising and deceptive food labels written in *legalese*?

Because more and more Americans are becoming health conscious, food and beverage manufacturers are trying to tap into this ever-growing market. They are reformulating their products in order to give them the appearance of legitimacy. Cadbury Schweppes is rolling out a reformulated 7up. They are labeling the new product "100% natural." The manufacturer has removed an artificial preservative and according to marketing vice-president Kelli Freeman, "... everything that remains in the can is from a natural source..." Don't be deceived by the phrase *from a natural source*. What this phrase really means is that you take something from nature, corn for instance, and then process it into high fructose corn syrup (HFCS). The executive director for the Center for Science in the Public Interest (CSPI), Michael Jacobson, says that "... high fructose corn syrup isn't something you could cook up from a bushel of corn in your kitchen, unless you happen to be equipped with centrifuges, hydroclones, ion-exchange columns, and buckets of enzymes..." High fructose corn syrup is not natural and is actually harmful to your health. Television ads show cans of 7up as fruits or veggies being plucked from the ground to emphasize their alleged 'naturalness.' This is deceptive advertising at its worse. I don't know about you, but it too is an insult to my intelligence.

Another claim you may find from food and beverage manufacturers peddling their 'natural' imitation wares is *naturally occurring*. Although a basic substance may be found in nature (naturally occurring), it does not mean that it is being used *in its natural state*! The ingredient being used started with something that is found in nature. The intensive processing that a *naturally occurring* substance undergoes makes it a health risk. Again we have a case of a claim perpetrated on the public with the intent to deceive.

If the FDA were to have a policy similar or identical to that of the USDA, Cadbury Schweppes' 7up couldn't be labeled as "100% natural." Not only would 7up be out of the running as an all natural product, but so would dozens of others.

100% ORGANIC

In October 2002 the USDA (United States Department of Agriculture) devised a standard policy for organic food. This policy does not allow the use of genetic engineering, ionizing radiation, sewage sludge, or several other substances in products bearing the organic label. There are four categories within the organic labeling family. 100 percent organic indicates that all ingredients must be totally organically produced.

ORGANIC

Food product must contain 95 percent or more organic ingredients.

MADE WITH ORGANIC INGREDIENTS

Product must have 70 to 95 percent organic ingredients.

PRODUCTS WITH LESS THAN 70% ORGANIC INGREDIENTS

Product ingredients must conform to defined organic regulations and product cannot bear the USDA seal.

IS THERE A MAGIC BULLET?

I guess its human nature to want to seek the path of least resistance. Let's face it, who wouldn't rather trek through mile high grass because it's a short cut as opposed to walking the long way around even though the long way is smooth and paved? Who wouldn't rather toss food into a microwave oven rather than stove cook it? You can't see it, but my hand is raised for the last question. I was guilty as charged. But what about taking a pharmaceutical pill to lose weight, or to prevent the body from absorbing fat from food eaten, as opposed to making a simple lifestyle change?

We all want to be able to have our cake, and eat it too. But there has always been a right way and a wrong way to do anything. Choose the wrong way and you will pay the price. This has often meant that we *couldn't* have our cake and eat it too. Decades ago the singer Gloria Taylor had a 45 vinyl record out called *You Got to Pay the Price*. How prophetic even when applied to health. Attempt to find a "magic bullet" and you *will* pay the price—a steep price. Concerning good nutrition and health, the right way is the *only* way to do it. When advising anyone about weight loss, I always tell them that they must work *with* the body, *not* against it. When God designed and made the body it was so perfect that no one, not even the food industry and their battery of top notch researchers and scientists, would be able to improve upon its maintenance. God's design calls for *natural* minerals, vitamins, fats, and other nutrients he specifically made for human consumption. There will *never* be a substitute.

One thing we must all keep in mind is that America is in the overweight and obesity epidemic war because it has abandoned physical activity and natural food choices. In their place Americans overindulge in muscle wasting and mind dulling activities such as video games and television, and polluting the body with synthetic chemicals masquerading as food.

When it comes to weight loss or reduction, the only way to work with the body is with a change in lifestyle. 'Magic bullets' such as fat blocking drugs are not an option, and never will be. These drugs are made by the pharmaceutical industry and they are totally synthetic. 'Synthetic' signifies toxic chemicals which will produce harmful side effects. And who knows what the long-term effect of these drugs will be? Not the Federal Drug Administration (FDA) or Big Pharma despite their claims and their tests.

The Saturday, April 8, 2006 edition of *The Star-Ledger*

reported that the fat-blocking drug in Xenical, a prescription form which received FDA approval in 1999, could be available later this year over-the-counter (OTC). Let it be understood that this fat-blocking drug will not affect the body fat a person is already carrying. But what it does is to block the fat digesting enzyme located in the gastrointestinal tract. This translates into about 1/3 of the fat in the food that you consume will not be digested. It will instead accumulate in the intestines and be passed out in the stool. The cost to the prospective consumer could reach up to $100 per month.

But there is a down side to this synthetic fat-blocking drug. It interferes with the body's absorption of the fat soluble vitamins A, D, E, K, and beta-carotene. And in the studies which have been conducted so far, the following side effects have occurred: *abdominal cramps, bloating, flatulence, increased bowel movements, and an inability to control them,* and what is being called *anal leakage.* Doesn't sound pretty does it? Some of the sleep drug commercials that I have seen on television warn that the person taking them shouldn't drive until the effects are known. A similar warning should be given to anyone taking fat-blocking drugs. "Don't go out in public until you know how you will be affected." Is that any way to live? And as I alluded to earlier, who knows what the far-ranging effects may be?

Other types of 'magic bullets' in the past have been *fat absorbing* drugs and *appetite suppressants.* Avoid anything that is produced by the pharmaceutical industry. Remember Fen-Phen? There are natural herbs and other substances available which are safe to take. But the best thing to do is exercise discipline and self-control when eating. The Bible says that there is nothing new under the sun. That truth has not changed even in this accelerated technological age. The majority of Americans managed to avoid being overweight or obese back when I was growing up. What has changed since that time has not been a natural occurrence, but a manufactured one.

God's way is the best and only way. With it you will lose those unwanted pounds of fat and maintain a lean and healthy body weight. There will be no short-term or long-term health issues and you won't waste money which could be better spent than by supporting the greedy and money hungry pharmaceutical industry.

OVERWEIGHT AND OBESITY INCREASING

Medical studies have shown that obesity increases the risk of type-2 diabetes by 300%, the risk of high cholesterol by 200%, the risk of heart disease by 200%, the risk of arthritis by 200%, and the risk of high blood pressure by 200%. There is also an increased risk of amputations, strokes, kidney failure, and blindness. 30% of the children in California are obese!

The war against an overweight and obese America must intensify. Right now we are losing it. At the moment, the leading cause of preventable death in America is tobacco. The second leading cause is poor diet and inactivity. A study has been released which says that if we don't start making head way in the war against obesity, deaths resulting from poor diet and physical inactivity will become the number one cause of preventable death in America. Since the last decade, deaths because of obesity and inactivity have risen by 33%.

In the year 2000, about 400,000 (17%) deaths were due to an unhealthy lifestyle. Deaths from tobacco in 2000 were 435,000. Medical scientists and researchers are constantly learning more and more about the negative effects of obesity. Doctors have already made the association between large waistlines and the increased risk of developing colorectal cancer, strokes, heart disease and diabetes. Now they are finding out that having excess body fat around the middle may affect the brain as well. Increased abdominal fat has been associated with brain changes which are linked to Alzheimer's disease.

Overweight and obesity know no color, religion, or nationality. Neither is there any distinction between rich and poor or Christian and non-Christian. I personally know of people who are no longer with us due to poor lifestyle choices. This is preventable. It doesn't have to be this way. The rich are overweight and obese from inactivity and their rich cuisine (rich in calories and price). The poor are overweight and obese from inactivity and their fast food cuisine. Everyone across the board would benefit from a positive lifestyle change.

In light of America's disturbing poor diet trend, we have to reexamine our eating habits. Are we eating to live or living to eat? God gave us a sense of taste so that we may enjoy eating nutritious food. We abuse that sense of taste when we continue destructive eating habits even when we become aware of them. The very first of God's Ten Commandments is, "Thou shalt have no other gods before me" (Exodus 20:3).

Food has become a god to so many people. *Anything* that controls is a god. The *"I can't live without. . . "* or *"I've got to have. . . "* mentality is a sign that there is a problem. Acknowledge it. Before a drug addict can be helped he must admit that he is a drug addict. Before an alcoholic can be helped, he must admit that he's an alcoholic. I mentioned the fact earlier that I love ice cream. I used to eat ice cream seven days a week. No kidding, I did. Even though I still worked out, that was a bit much. I decided that I wanted to lose the extra fat from around my waist and lower back. In order to achieve my goal of getting my waistline from 37 inches to 32 inches or under I had to give up the ice cream. Did I say, "I can't do it?" or "I'm not giving it up?" No I didn't. *I simply gave it up!* I maintain my waist now at less than 33 inches.

I never did like the idea of anything controlling me—*anything at all!* The only one that should control your life is the Holy Spirit. Before I became born again I used to drink and smoke cigarettes and marijuana. The friends I was hanging out with did the same. But as time went on they became more deeply involved in the alcohol. They also progressed to other drugs, and various pills. Two of them died as an indirect result of this lifestyle choice. Subconsciously I never wanted anything to so totally possess me that I was helpless and had no control. I stopped drinking and gave up smoking cigarettes and marijuana.

Unlike marijuana or cocaine or any other illegal drug, there is no negative stigma attached to poor food choices. But in order to help those who are finding it difficult to change bad food choices, play the following mind game. Imagine that making bad food choices are like taking an illegal drug. Not only is it detrimental to the body, but pretend that it is against the law also. Fight the urge or inclination to eat fast and processed food. You are going to "kick the habit." Come on, you can do it.

I don't want poor eating habits to control my life. Although I have eaten clean for the last few years (foods consistent with maintaining a healthy and lean physique), I have recently made the choice to eat everything 100% organic. When it comes to my health, and avoiding hospitals and drugs, no one has to preach to me. I will *never* be dependent on prescription or nonprescription drugs. Nor will I finance a doctor's dream house. Neither will I ever be an overweight, flabby and weak person. I will continue to exercise by lifting weights well into my 90s or 100s depending on how long God permits me to live. Hey, I'm serious!

Choices. We all have choices—lifestyle choices. I choose to do it God's way so that I can enjoy the maximum benefits in my Christian walk. This is the mind set that you have to adopt. There was a disco song out in the 70s called *Ain't No Stopping Us Now.* My eyes have been opened. God's Word has revealed what He wants for His people. Nothing will prevent me from having it. There *ain't no stopping me now.*

You too can live an overcoming and abundant Christian life. Choose not to be a part of that escalating poor eating statistic. God has an investment in you. Jesus died to save you from your sins. But He also died so that you could fulfill your mission on earth. In order to do that you must be healthy and fit. You must commit to reclaiming the body that God has so much invested in, along with the spirit and soul.

Fully realizing God's investment in you will transcend any selfish desires on your part. The Bible says that we are not our own—that we were bought with a price (I Corinthians 6:19–20). We are to glorify God in our bodies. I am not talking about narcissism or self-love. What I am talking about is self-respect—respect for the body which God indwells by His Holy Spirit. Back in the 70s, the Staple Singers had a song on the charts called *Respect Yourself.* Respecting the 'temple of the Holy Ghost' means loving and cherishing what God has created. This translates to proper nutrition and exercise in the physical realm.

Weight gain, or loss for that matter, seems to first show in a person's face. I know years ago when I dieted for a bodybuilding competition, my face would appear thinner. I have just started noticing the unhealthy weight gain in peoples' faces which comes from eating too much fast food. The face gets plumper. As the face goes, so does the rest of the body. This plumpness is not reflective of the healthy and normal weight gain. It is the kind which comes from the hormones with which cattle are injected, and the trans fats and MSG and other deadly chemicals found in fast foods. Unfortunately this plumpness is a precursor to certain types of cancer, high blood pressure, diabetes, and other potential life threatening diseases.

BENZENE AND SOFT DRINKS

Parents who are concerned about what their children are drinking have filed class action lawsuits against the soft drink companies, Polar Beverages and In Zone Brands. Polar Beverages bottles sodas, seltzers, mixers and water; In Zone Brands manufactures the BellyWashers line of sugar laden juice drinks. The lawsuit claims that these companies had inadequate procedures for ensuring that the chemical benzene did not become a part of their products.

Benzene is a carcinogen (cancer-causing agent) which is used in the production of plastics, detergents, and pesticides. It is produced naturally by the burning of natural products. Benzene has caused leukemia to develop in people who have been exposed to it. Even short-term exposure to high quantities of benzene can be deadly.

The Federal Drug Administration (FDA) has found that out of the soft drinks they have sampled, 80% contained benzene levels four times greater than that present in tap water! The maximum allowable limit of benzene that our water supply can contain is 5 parts per billion according to the Environmental Protection Agency (EPA). Benzene can form in soft drinks made with vitamin C and either sodium benzoate or potassium benzoate. Other factors such as heat and light and the length of time these soft drinks sit on store shelves also influence the formation of benzene.

Here is another reason to eliminate all soft drinks from the diet. The FDA knew almost 15 years ago that ascorbic acid and sodium benzoate or potassium benzoate are able to form the deadly benzene upon a chemical reaction. They then left it up to the soft drink industry to take care of the problem. It seems to me that if the Food and Drug Administration is an agency which is responsible for the welfare of the public, they should have exerted their authority and insist the industry eliminate the problem—or at least make sure the levels of benzene were at an acceptable level (if there is an acceptable level for poison).

Neither the FDA nor any other federal agency is concerned about the public welfare. Given the facts of the situation, it is up to the individual to decide a course of action. All soft drinks, whether regular or diet, contain high fructose corn syrup and other obesity producing sugars. They don't provide any nutrition for the body. Neither to they quench the thirst. Since God made our bodies approximately 66% water, He intended for us to drink water, not processed chemicals which taste good.

With all the soft drinks that are consumed today, I would dare say that a majority of Americans are not drinking enough pure water (water by itself). The body should be hydrated at all times. At least eight, 8 ounce glasses of water should be drunk on a daily basis. More if you are physically active. By the way, don't just drink water when you are thirsty. Thirst itself is not a good indicator. An indicator of a properly hydrated body is the color of the urine. If it is a pale yellow, you are properly hydrated. If your urine is a dark yellow, or worse, different shades of orange, you are not drinking nearly enough.

Drinking enough pure water is yet another step in living a God-glorifying life through good health. So drink up!

SUBSTANCE ABUSE

I have already listed the foods, and various chemicals and sugars and fats that should be avoided. What many consumers do not realize, including myself until recently, is that their strong influence on us can be classified as *substance abuse*. We are all familiar with alcohol, nicotine, and illegal drugs. But what we don't realize is that food and soft drink companies include ingredients in their products for the express purpose of getting the consumer "hooked" on them. The monosodium glutamate (MSG) and the high fructose corn syrup (HFCS) and all the other sugars and fats that I have explained are included in foods and soft drinks to captivate the taste buds. Once these products have been tasted, and a "taste" has been acquired for them, they are hard to resist.

I remember once a few years back I was discussing with my students the problem of being overweight and how the foods we love to eat influenced it. They remarked that it was the fats in these foods which made them taste so good. They were right. But it isn't just the fats in the processed food; sugars also play a large role. And the food companies who want to have you as a lifelong consumer of their products invested time and money in finding the right chemicals to mix into their products. These chemicals are designed to make you fat and to get you addicted. After a while, like a junkie needing a "fix," it gets to the point that you've got to have the fries, soft drinks, the burgers, and all the other processed foods which are *nutritionally challenged.*

Like alcohol, nicotine, sniffing glue and all the other chemical abuses which entrap the unwary, the processed foods and soft drinks which contain chemical additives are dangerous to the body and mind. This is what makes the abuse so dangerous—the destructiveness to one's health by opening the door to potentially life threatening medical problems. Once that door is opened, and high blood pressure or high cholesterol or heart disease results, the typical solution to these and other conditions is synthetic prescription and nonprescription drugs which themselves can cause other serious medical problems.

The substance abuse of refined carbohydrates and processed

foods is as great as, or greater than any danger posed by alcohol or tobacco. God does not want our minds enslaved and our bodies destroyed by these foreign chemicals. Our bodies are resilient and are able to fight off many foreign invaders. But there comes a point where the natural defenses are so overwhelmed by synthetic drugs that they completely decimate both body and mind. This is the point where behavior becomes decidedly more hostile, and various cancers or heart disease or stroke appear, and multiply.

WHAT THE MEAT AND DAIRY INDUSTRIES DON'T WANT YOU TO KNOW

"And God said, Let us make man in our image, after our likeness: and let them have dominion over the fish of the sea, and over the fowl of the air, and over the cattle, and over all the earth, and over every creeping thing that creepeth upon the earth" (Genesis 1:26).

God created man to manage the earth, and to rule over every living creature on it. Man has been given the responsibility by his Creator to care for the animal creation. This responsibility does not include running roughshod over the animals and treating them with hatred and contempt. Like man, animals respond to, and need, love. Although God has also given man the right to use animal and marine life for food, that right does not include abusing or torturing the animal in the process. Unfortunately the modern meat and dairy industries have abused God's mandate to man by mistreating animals that are to be killed for food. Even animals scheduled for our lunch and dinner plates ought to be treated with some amount of dignity and a lot of care.

Driven by the love of money, the meat and dairy industries employ any and all methods to process cows, chickens, turkeys, and pigs at minimum cost. The methods follow after the pattern of the modern day factory and employ assembly line techniques. And like the factory, the animals are treated as though they were manufactured, unfeeling, inanimate objects instead of living, breathing creatures. The animals are not allowed to graze as God designed them to. They are removed from their natural environment and confined in extremely tight quarters. There was a time when chickens, pigs, and turkeys were raised on farms. They were allowed to move around and graze. Not any more. Instead of being farm raised, it is more accurate to say that they are factory-raised.

Cows are used for one of two purposes: meat or milk. Their purpose dictates to an extent in what manner they are treated. Neither treatment is good. If the cow is to be used for meat, they are typically allowed to spend the first year of their lives grazing. Prior to 1950, all cattle had the luxury of grazing in the open as God intended for them to do. By the 1970s, this practice was a thing of the past.

Cows to be used for meat often freeze to death in the winter and others fall victim to heat stroke in the summertime. Veterinary care for them is scarce, if at all. The cows who survive this ordeal are auctioned off. They are then shipped to huge feedlots where they are crammed together like sardines in a can. The journey, however, leaves many of them crippled while others die. Cows are shipped to feedlots in trucks. Out of every 100 shipped, one dies from a form of pneumonia known as *shipping fever*. To fight this disease, the animals are given an antibiotic called chloramphenicol. This is a powerful drug which can kill humans who are susceptible to it. Trace or residual amounts of this deadly drug remain even after the animal is slaughtered, and thus enters the human food chain.

God made cows to eat grass. Cows in these cramped factory style feedlots are fed just about anything but grass. Cattlemen need to get the cows as fat as possible in the shortest amount of time possible. And of course, cost is a factor. ". . . Cattle raised for food are also pumped full of drugs to make them grow faster and keep them alive in these miserable conditions. . . Many feedlot owners simply give the animals even higher doses of human-grade antibiotics in an attempt to keep them alive long enough to make it to the slaughterhouse. . ."[49]

Remember, a cow's natural diet is grass. These poor creatures however are fed sawdust mixed with ammonia, shredded newspaper (these are not goats people, they are cows), processed sewage, and other unspeakable inedible garbage, along with man's finest chemical concoctions known as insecticides, antibiotics and synthetic hormones! This trash causes the cow severe digestive pain. Some internal organs become ulcerated and actually burst from the trauma. As much as 32% of cows "groomed" for beef develop potentially fatal liver abscesses.

Trace amounts of deadly antibiotics and insecticides are stored in animals, and only a handful of animal carcasses are ever tested for chemical poisons. Only a small percentage of the known poisons in America's meat supply are actually tested for. The majority of meat destined for consumers fall through the USDA's cracks.

Cows raised for their milk get no better treatment than those raised for beef. They are treated as though they were simply money generating machines. Cows which are destined for milk production are constantly sick and diseased just as those used for meat because their environment is highly unsanitary. The odors of their urine and feces which they have to stand in are stifling.

Milk cows are continuously impregnated. The calves are taken away from their mothers within a day of their birth. The female calves will share the same fate as their mothers. The males are destined to wind up as veal. Immediately after birth, the mother cows are connected up to milking machines. Injected with bovine growth hormone (BGH), these cows produce up to ten times the milk as is natural! (By the way, BGH has been banned in Canada and Europe due to concerns of human health and the cow's welfare. America doesn't care). This tortuous process causes a painful inflammation of the cow's udder known as *mastitis*. According to the dairy industry's own statistics, approximately 30% to 50% of milking cows fall prey to mastitis.

The average life span for a cow is 25 years. Dairy cows however live only 1/5 that time. You have to keep in mind that the hamburger meat or veal or milk that you consume don't come from healthy cows. Their abusive treatment and grossly unsanitary environment prevents good health from being even a remote possibility. What does this mean to you the consumer? Before slaughter or death, the cow is diseased and has been fed what no one in his right mind would call food. It is certainly not what God created it to eat. To combat their disease and other crippling health issues, cows are pumped full of antibiotics. They are also injected with the hormone BGH. This is not to mention the insecticides and herbicides which they ingest.

Science and medicine have limitations. While man continues to bring new innovations, inventions, medical procedures, and drugs to the market, he cannot possibly anticipate what may come about in time because of an invention or medical procedure; neither can he predict how a patient or consumer will respond when drugs are taken under varying conditions. For example, the food industry didn't know that their introduction of trans fatty acids into foods would be worse in terms of health than the saturated fat which the consumer didn't want anymore.

Traces of the hormones, insecticides, herbicides, pesticides, and antibiotics remain in the meat and in the milk that is marketed. This is contributing to America's health crisis and the rise in various cancers. You are literally playing Russian roulette with non-organic meat and milk products. Remember the saying *you are what you eat*. This is literally true. You are eating meat from diseased cows, pigs, chickens, and turkeys. You are drinking milk from diseased cows. You are also feeding your body synthetic chemical compounds—*deadly* synthetic chemical compounds. 80% of salmonellosis (caused by salmonella and resulting in fever, malaise, and intestinal disorders) in human beings originate in diseased animal food. This is a formula for disaster, not for building a healthy, God-glorifying body. "...Dr. Egger reminds us that low concentrations of antibiotics are measurable in many of our foods, rivers, and streams around the world. Much of this is seeping into bodies of water from animal farms..."[50]

The number of adults being diagnosed with cancer is rising. I had always wondered what the cause of cancer besides cigarette smoking was. Now I know. Indoor and outdoor pollution (including second-hand smoke) and the chemicals that we eat and drink along with our water, milk, and meats are primary factors. The incubation period for cancer is years. Food and milk processing have undergone changes over the last 50 or so years. Unfortunately these changes have not been for the better. I daresay that the food and dairy industries have seen these changes as the implementation of new technology, and better and faster ways of doing things. But, if new technology, and better and faster leads to deteriorating quality and unhealthy products, they cannot be justified. And since the meat and dairy industries do not have a monopoly on their products, the public does not have to consume what the food and dairy industry decides to put on the market in the name of profit. The new innovations started a chain of events which would result in various types of cancer in ever increasing numbers. As food consumption has been on the rise, more and more carcinogens are being ingested. This is leading to greater numbers of people being diagnosed with cancer.

THE TRUTH ABOUT BOTTLED WATER

Bottled water has become mainstream. Every food mart, convenience store, and supermarket carries it. Not only do professional athletes and week-end athletes swear by it, but so does the ordinary housewife and college student. Bottled water is an alternative to municipal tap water. Filtered water is the other alternative. It seems as though hardly anyone trusts municipal water anymore. Americans purchased bottled water in the staggering amount of $7 billion dollars in 2003. 6.8 billion gallons of bottled water are consumed in America every year. In general, bottled water is more expensive than ordinary tap water. The bottled water mania is not confined to America either, it is worldwide.

Of course bottled water did not exist when I was growing up. Our only source back then was the tap water we received from the kitchen faucet. What generated the market for bottled water? The one incident which may have heavily influenced the amazing growth of the bottled water industry happened in Milwaukee, Wisconsin in the spring of 1993. An outbreak of cryptosporidium, a waterborne disease, infected more than 400,000 city residents. In 1976 cryptosporidium was identified in humans. And in following years this disease was found almost exclusively in

AIDS victims. Cryptosporidium attacks the gastrointestinal tract of those infected. It was on the morning of April 5, 1993 that the Milwaukee Health Department received numerous phone calls from residents and from the news media. The complaint was gastrointestinal distress. Water was almost immediately suspected.

Believe it or not but bottled water is defined as a 'food' under federal regulations. As such it is regulated by the Food and Drug Administration (FDA). Tap water on the other hand is not identified as a 'food' and is therefore under the regulations of the Environmental Protection Agency (EPA). EPA regulations are much more stringent than FDA regulations.

Is bottled water all that it is cracked up to be? Crucial to leading a God-glorifying life through good health is being able to drink pure and uncontaminated water. Clearly the possibility of tap water becoming infected is there. We have already shown in Chapter 1 that tap water is chlorinated and fluoridated by the water company. Chlorine and fluoride are deadly poisons. We definitely need an alternative to tap water. It is therefore important that bottled water be as contaminant free as possible.

It has come out in the media that Coca-Cola has been less than honest in promoting its bottled water, Dasani. Dasani had been advertised as originating from natural springs. In actuality, Coca-Cola had been getting the water from the water companies and then purifying it. Purification notwithstanding, Coca-Cola lied. What other deceptions are they perpetrating on the public? What about other bottled water? Can they be trusted? Keep in mind that the bottled water industry is worldwide and is worth billions of dollars. The Bible says that the love of money is the root of all evil. When this kind of money is involved, false promotions will run rampant.

The National Resources Defense Council (nrdc) undertook a four-year study of bottled water. They published their findings in 1999. Of the more than 1,000 samples of 103 brands of bottled water tested, 25% or more was just ordinary tap water. Sometimes the tap water was treated, and other times it was not. One particular brand of bottled water was advertised as 'spring water.' It was found to have been pumped from a water source adjacent to a hazardous waste dumping site. And as if that wasn't bad enough, the nrdc study also discovered that one fifth of the brands of bottled water it looked at tested positive for industrial chemicals and other chemicals such as phthalate. Phthalate seeps into bottled water from its plastic container. This chemical interferes with sex hormone receptors. What other harm will they be found to cause in the coming years?

Since bottled water falls under the looser standards of the FDA, it may be less safe than tap water—depending on the brand. The companies which sell bottled water are under no mandate to give a detailed account of the water's origin and contaminant level violations, if any. Whereas municipal water systems have to test for microbiological infestation several times a day, bottled water companies only have to test *once a week*. The companies who sell bottled water are not required to test for cryptosporidium, the chlorine resistant protozoan that affected the residents of Milwaukee, Wisconsin in 1993.

I have given you the facts and it is up to you what to do with them. To date I haven't fallen prey to bottled water. I still drink tap water. Given the results of my research, I think tap water is the lesser of the two evils. It is certainly less expensive. But I am in the process of purchasing a home water filter system. My research has shown that of all the purification methods, filtration is best. Water filtration removes more deadly contaminants than any other process. It is designed to work especially with municipal water systems. Unlike bottled water and tap water, after tap water is filtered, if any cryptosporidium is present, it is removed.

Go to web site www.allaboutwater.org to learn all about water.

DECEITFUL MEAT

"When thou sittest to eat with a ruler, *consider diligently* what is before thee: And put a knife to thy throat, if thou be a man *given to appetite*. Be not desirous of his dainties: for they are *deceitful meat*" (Proverbs 23:1–3).

In an earlier chapter I told you a piece of wisdom that was given to my classmates and me by our high school chemistry teacher. He told us that, "A word to the wise is sufficient." I have never forgotten that. If you recall your Bible, upon his request Solomon was given wisdom from God. It was Solomon who penned the scriptures above, as well as the entire book of Proverbs.

Notice the three phrases that I italicized above: *consider diligently*, *given to appetite*, and *deceitful meat*. Since Solomon used the phrase *consider diligently*, what he is about to say is very important. To be diligent involves painstaking effort and care. We are to carefully pay attention to the foods that are in front of us. Obviously we shouldn't eat everything. *Given to appetite* implies someone who lets his stomach do his thinking. This person is at a disadvantage. He loves to eat. And he will eat what his passions dictate despite any consequences. Listen to what Paul says in Philippians 3:19. "*Whose end is destruction, whose God is their belly, and whose glory is in their shame, who mind earthly things.*" If you, despite cautions and warnings, and health risks, stubbornly continue to eat foods which harm your body, then your god is your belly. Exodus 20:5 says that God is a jealous God.

The grave is full of Christians who ignored doctor's and concerned family members' warnings, and maybe even those of the pastor, to give up eating certain foods for health's sake. Sad to say, their belly was their god. And how many Christians go to the altar Sunday after Sunday for prayer for some health condition? Many times the chronic health problems stem from poor eating habits and food choices. The simplistic belief that the devil is behind every ache and pain, or cancer or high blood pressure is simply not true. The Holy Spirit will let those prayer warriors who are sensitive to His Spirit know what's behind all illnesses brought to the altar.

Everyone who goes to the altar for healing doesn't need a miracle. What is needed is a word of wisdom from the Holy Spirit to stop drinking all of that soda, or to stop eating all that fried food, or maybe give up the nutrition less white bread, white rice, white sugar, and white table salt. I personally know of one person who had severe health issues, and had been told that by a doctor. Despite the doctor's strict diet, this person continued to eat forbidden foods. That proved to be a death wish.

The last phrase of Proverbs 23:3 is *deceitful meat*. The foods most destructive to the health are highly processed and refined. They are engineered by food companies to appeal to the eyes, nose (smell), and taste. No one has to tell me that Burger King's *Big Mac* looks, smells, and tastes good. I know from experience. It is the palate's delight. But it is 'deceitful meat.' The Big Mac is high in fat, salt, and sugar. 'Deceitful meat' is one of Satan's most masterful tactics. He has ensnared more seasoned Christians with this device than by almost any other. Food is a sore point with many people. Many will become defensive when confronted with this satanic strategy.

Unfortunately in today's world, food that you would not ordinarily think of as being bad for your health is. Non organic meat, non organic fruits and vegetables, and non organic dairy products are not as safe as they were in great grandfather's day. Our meats are laden with deadly hormones and antibiotics. Fruits and vegetables are saturated with herbicides and insecticides. The body was not designed by God to absorb them. These toxins are the root cause of various cancers, diabetes, heart diseases, multiple sclerosis, and dozens of other debilitating health problems. Nothing is safe anymore. Not even fish from the depths of the ocean. They haven't escaped man's unwise and runaway technology. Mercury is the number one worry with fish. That's bad enough. But are there other poisons in fish that we don't know of? I dread to even think about it.

Gillis Triplett of Gillis Triplett Ministries tells the following story. The Holy Spirit sent him to a couple in the apartment complex where he lived when he first moved to Georgia. He had a word of knowledge concerning their appetites. Both husband and wife rejected what Gillis told them about their passion for eating certain foods. About a year afterwards, the husband asked Gillis to pray for his wife who was only twenty-eight years old. She had contracted multiple sclerosis. The Holy Spirit revealed to Gillis that the wife hadn't had a bowel movement in over a month. He told the husband to tell that to the doctors. He was also told to tell the doctors not to prescribe any medication to aid in bowel movements. In over a little more than a year later, the wife was completely bedridden. Husband and wife still rejected Gillis' health warning. After another year passed, the husband wanted prayer for himself for what he thought was pink eye. The Holy Spirit let Gillis know that the husband's problem was more serious than just pink eye. He told the husband this. When he went to the hospital it was discovered that the husband had a brain aneurysm. It was found in the nick of time. Gillis remarked that husband and wife could have avoided their health issues if they had obeyed the Holy Spirit concerning eating certain foods.[51]

You are thinking to yourself, "I hear what you're saying. But what if I pray over my food before I eat it?" Well it's good that you bless your food before eating it. Remember that person I mentioned above who didn't adhere to the doctor's diet? Well that person told me directly that he prayed over his forbidden food before it was eaten. Despite the prayers, he succumbed to the health problems brought upon by the toxic food. God does not bless anyone who willingly ignores truth. To think that God will nullify toxic food effects just because you prayed over it is like believing that God would spare your life if, despite being warned, you drove your car over a road whose bridge had collapsed. Just because you prayed before leaving home doesn't mean that God will miraculously support your car through empty space until you reached the other side. You willingly drove down that road having been told that its bridge was out. God is not a magic genie.

The average consumer is at a distinct disadvantage when it comes to the food, dairy, and pharmaceutical industries. These industries have an army of scientists, lawyers, and advertisers to do one thing. That is to get you, the consumer, to purchase their products, and to be a loyal customer of those products. Billions of dollars are at stake and these industries will do anything to keep their coffers full. Your health is not their concern. If you are not committed to, and take responsibility for your health, believe me, no one else will. Don't grieve the Holy Spirit by neglecting your health. The dangerous foods that you eat are not that important. Believe what I tell you from experience. You can still enjoy eating by including only organic products on your menu. And I guarantee that you will be a whole lot healthier.

OBESITY AND BODY TYPE

Generally speaking, an individual's body shape follows one of two basic patterns. There is the "apple" shape and the "pear" shape. A person having an "apple" shaped body type carries fat predominately around the waist (the abdominal region). A pear-shaped body type carries fat mostly around the hips.

A method used to help determine body fat levels along with BMI (body mass index) is the waist-to-hip ratio. One study found that the waist-to-hip ratio was the most accurate indicator of heart attack risk. To find your ratio you need a tape measure. Measure your waist and your hips. Now divide the waist measurement by the hip measurement. As an example, my waist measures 33 inches while my hips measures 39 inches. I simply divide 33 inches by 39 inches. My waist-to-hip ratio is 0.85. A woman's waist-to-hip ratio should be 0.8 or less; a man's ratio should be anywhere from 0.95 to 1.0 or less (depending on who you talk to). Ratios greater than numbers given above puts the individual at increased risk for heart disease, diabetes, and certain types of cancer. This also signifies that the person has an apple body type. Excess abdominal body fat (apple) elevates the risk for all types of health problems. ". . . People who carry weight in the 'metabolically active' abdomen are at higher risk for heart disease and diabetes than those who pack their pounds in the butt and thighs. Okay, so you have no control over where those pesky pounds reside. . ."[52]

Nobody has to sit back and let the devil make their body a ticking time bomb, or hang a death sentence around their neck. A God-glorifying life in good health is yours for the taking. Note I said "taking," not "asking." Satan has sabotaged your health with a well thought out and subtle plan. He has enlisted the support of the food and dairy industries to produce tempting tasty delights for you to eat yourself into an early grave. God wants you to "take back" your health by force (Read Matthew 11:12).

He has empowered you to do it too. Knowledge is the key. This book provides the knowledge. All you have to do is implement it. Before I began the research for this book, I was ignorant of the conscious effort of the pharmaceutical, food, and dairy industries to get America addicted to their health destroying products. I am ignorant no longer, and neither are you.

A lifestyle change encompassing nutrition and exercise is the only way to break the enemy's stranglehold on a seemingly oblivious American public. There are no shortcuts. And there is no other way.

IRRADIATED FOODS

The latest technology employed to ensure food safety is called *irradiation*. This process uses low radiation levels to destroy harmful microbes such as salmonella and E. coli. Currently there are three radiation methods:

1. Gamma rays
2. X-rays and
3. Electron beams

Irradiation was approved by the FDA (Food and Drug Administration) in 1997. The USDA (United States Department of Agriculture) approved the sale of irradiated products in grocery stores in 1999. Irradiation can be used for meats, fruits, and vegetables.

Although the FDA assures us that thorough testing on animals and humans was performed, who knows what the long-term effect may be? Everyone thought that microwaving foods was safe too. The FDA says that radiation isn't absorbed by the food and there is only a small loss of nutrients.

Man is again using technology to process food which will ultimately wind up in our stomachs. I don't want to be repetitious, but again I must stress that although no short-term effects were observed, scientists and doctors are unable to predict what the long-term results may be. It may be that some people will experience an allergic reaction to it. They just don't know. God's original menu is best. Buy organic meats, fruits and vegetables and you will not have to worry about irradiation. It was man who placed himself into such a dire situation where harmful microbes and insects are such a threat that extreme measures such as irradiation have to be resorted to.

Foods that have been irradiated have to be labeled as such. This symbol

indicates that the product has been treated with radiation. You should avoid all irradiated products in order to live a God-glorifying life through good health. Your health is much too precious to leave to chance and to man whose overriding concern is profit.

CHAPTER 5:

Good For Food

INTRODUCTION

"And God said, Behold, I have given you *every herb bearing seed*, which is upon the face of all the earth, *and every tree, in the which is the fruit of a tree yielding seed*; to you it shall be for meat" (Genesis 1:29).

"And out of the ground made the Lord God to grow every tree that is pleasant to the sight, and *good for food*; the tree of life also in the midst of the garden, and the tree of knowledge of good and evil" (Genesis 2:9).

"Every moving thing that liveth shall be meat for you; even as the green herb have I given you all things" (Genesis 9:3).

God originally created man as a total vegetarian (also known as *vegan*). He was an herbivore. This means that his original diet consisted of fruits, vegetables, legumes (dried beans and peas), grains (rice, wheat), seeds and nuts. As a matter of fact, every land animal was vegan too. This included but was not limited to lions, tigers, dinosaurs, bears, etc. "Meat" in Genesis 1:29 and 9:3 means "food."

Everything that man needed for growth and sustenance was provided for through plant life. Protein, carbohydrates, fats, minerals and vitamins were complete and in abundance in the lush and luxurious green plants and trees in the Garden of Eden. We can only speculate about the almost endless variety of fruits, vegetables, grains, and beans that were located there. And there was no sin present to mar the environment or the food.

It is quite apparent that if Adam had not sinned, man's diet would yet be *every herb bearing seed* and *every tree*. Originally he was not permitted to hunt land animals or to fish for marine life. Hunting and fishing meant death—for the animal and fish that is. Death signifies sin. "Wherefore, as by one man sin entered into the world, and death by sin; and so death passed upon all men, for that all have sinned" (Romans 5:12). Death was the inevitable result of man's sin. It will be banished in the future. "And God shall wipe away all tears from their eyes; and there shall be *no more death*, neither sorrow, nor crying, neither shall there be any more pain: for the former things are passed away" (Revelation 21:4). The phrase *no more death* is not qualified to signify man only. *There will be no death of any living creature.*

After Adam's sin and after the worldwide flood, God permitted man to incorporate animals into his diet. Both diets were healthy and provided optimum nutrition. Of course there was no engineered food back then. Everything was 100 percent organic. And unlike today, animals roamed freely (grazed) and ate perfectly nutritious vegetation.

The Bible intimates that God may return man and animal to a vegetarian diet during Christ's millennial reign. "And the cow and the bear shall feed; their young ones shall lie down together: and the lion *shall eat straw* like the ox" (Isaiah 11:7). The same seems to be true for the eternal age also. It is hard to imagine man slaughtering animals for meat during this time. "In the midst of the street of it, and on either side of the river, was there the tree of life, *which bare twelve manner of fruits, and yielded her fruit every month*: and the leaves of the tree were for the healing of the nations" (Revelation 22:2).

DANIEL WAS VEGAN

Of course everything changed as a result of man's sin and the subsequent flood. For one thing, God cursed the ground from which grew plants, trees, and grains—man's entire vegetarian diet. "And unto Adam he said, Because thou hast hearkened unto the voice of thy wife, and hast eaten of the tree, of which I commanded thee, saying, Thou shalt not eat of it: *cursed is the ground* for thy sake; in sorrow shalt thou eat of it all the days of thy life" (Genesis 3:17).

Though cursed, the earth still provided nutritious vegetation. It was nothing like we have today. The soil was yet fertile and free of chemical pollutants. Daniel led a vegan life.

Although it's hard to believe that a Hebrew would pass up a meal consisting of roasted lamb chops, Daniel chose to. "But Daniel purposed in his heart that he would not defile himself with the portion of the king's meat, nor with the wine which he drank: therefore he requested of the prince of the eunuchs that he might not defile himself" (Daniel 1:8).

Daniel was also a teetotaler. He refused to drink wine. Daniel's entire diet consisted of foods of plant and vegetable origin, and water. He specifically asked for pulse (the edible seeds of peas, beans, lentils). Obviously this diet was healthier than that of the Babylonians because Daniel and his companions appeared healthier.

VEGETARIAN DIET

Is a vegetarian diet healthier for you than a diet which includes meat? Vegans and vegetarians would obviously answer in the affirmative while those who include meat in their diets would say "no way, Jose." There is overwhelming evidence however that a vegetarian diet is the healthiest diet of them all. I was not always a vegetarian. I did though restrict my meat consumption to poultry such as chicken and turkey breasts (all organic of course). But I was always open-minded, and willing to try something new. With all things considered, and having searched through the biblical record, it seems that God's perfect will was for man to be an herbivore. Let us not forget, originally man was created an herbivore. Biblical evidence strongly suggests that man will return to his vegetarian roots.

One of the longest living societies on the face of the earth is the Hunzas. Their diet consists almost exclusively of fruits, vegetables, and grain. They eat very little meat. There are two other groups who enjoy longer than average life spans, the Vilcambas of the Andes Mountains of Ecuador and the Abkhasians of the Black Sea area of Russia. Their diets also are almost entirely vegetarian.

I think Americans consume too much red meat. It is high in saturated fat and cholesterol. There have been many studies done on vegetarian versus non-vegetarian diets. They almost all show that vegetarians have a lower risk of obesity, coronary heart disease, high blood pressure, and certain forms of cancer than their meat eating counterparts. A Yale study has shown that a diet high in red meat (saturated fat), eggs and dairy products results in an increased risk of Non-Hodgkin's Lymphoma, a cancer of the lymphatic system. At the same time this study has shown that a diet high in veggies such as broccoli, tomatoes and others reduce the risk of this particular form of cancer by 40%. This research was reported in the *American Journal of Epidemiology*.[53]

Another problem with red meat is that it is a source of iron. The body needs iron but too much can be toxic. Iron, along with copper and aluminum, generate free radicals. This results in premature aging, cancer, diabetes, atherosclerosis, and neurodegenerative diseases. People who eat red meat every day have a much higher risk of these serious diseases than people who do not. Studies have shown that women who eat a hamburger every day incur a 300% increase in the risk of developing breast cancer.

However vegetables high in iron do not pose a health risk. This is because vegetables also contain flavonoids which do not allow excess iron to be absorbed into the body.

Pulse and legumes have been around for centuries. As we have seen, Daniel ate them. Archeologists have discovered these vegetables in ancient towns of the eastern Mediterranean and in Mesopotamia and even in Egyptian pyramids. Beans and all the other legumes are high in complex carbohydrates, protein, fiber, and low in fat. They are important in the fight against heart disease, cancer, and obesity.

Studies have shown that lacto-ovo vegetarians (who eat dairy products and eggs) have 1/3 the heart disease mortality rates of those who eat meat. Strict vegetarians experience only 1/10 the death rate from heart disease as do meat eaters. The *American Journal of Clinical Nutrition* reported this amazing study which involved 24,000 people. The evidence is overwhelming and incontrovertible.

The June, 2006 issue of *Reader's Digest* printed the following in its Health IQ section: "Switching to a vegetarian diet can help prevent weight gain." A vegetarian diet doesn't have the saturated fat found in a meat diet.

NON-VEGETARIAN DIET

When I included meat in my diet, I did regulate what kinds of meat I ate. I had given up eating red meat (I did have a lean cut of steak occasionally though). I ate organic chicken breasts and turkey breasts. You may not realize it but cows are fed and raised contrary to their nature. They should be allowed to roam free and eat grass. Instead they are confined and fed ground up and diseased animals, and pumped full of hormones and antibiotics. If you do choose to eat red meat, *organic is a must*.

Several studies indicate that the consumption of red meat causes DNA damage to colon cells which in turn raises the risk of developing colon cancer. A comprehensive 20 year study conducted by the American Cancer Society (ACS) found that people who eat read meat, whether beef, pork, lamb, or processed meat, get colon cancer 30% to 40% more often than those who eat red meat occasionally. It is even worse for people who eat a lot of the luncheon meats such as hot dogs, sausages, and salami. The risk of developing colon cancer is 50%.

Eating more fruit and vegetables is also a must. The average American eats only 3 servings of fruit and vegetables a day. This is totally inadequate. Nutritionists are now saying that we should be eating anywhere from 5 to 13 servings of fruit and vegetables a day (the exact serving size depends on your specific caloric requirement). Remember your mother telling you to "eat your vegetables?" She was right.

We all should increase our intake of fruit and vegetables. Not only is the number of servings important, but variety is too. Consume a wide variety of fruit and veggies. A diet high in fruit and vegetables has been found to fight against cancer, heart disease, stroke, high blood pressure, high cholesterol and promotes gastrointestinal health and good vision. No wonder God placed man on a vegetarian diet.

COOKING MEATS AT HIGH TEMPERATURES

There have been studies which show that meats cooked at high temperatures (well done) produces carcinogens (cancer causing agents) despite the method of cooking (frying, BBQ, broiling, etc). In general, cooking meats at high temperatures for a long period of time is potentially hazardous to the health. This is due to certain carcinogens which are formed in the process.

A study which was presented at a meeting of the American Association for Cancer Research shows that there is a link between meats cooked at high temperatures and a higher risk of men developing prostate cancer. A compound called PhIP, a carcinogen, is formed when meat is cooked at very high temperatures such as is produced when grilling or barbecuing. Another group of carcinogens that have been identified with meat cooked at high temperatures is called *heterocyclic amines*.

Studies also indicate an increased risk of breast cancer in women who ate meats cooked at high temperatures, especially by barbecuing or broiling. There was double the risk in women who ate meats cooked at high temperatures compared with women who ate meats cooked at a lower temperature. Charring of meats on grills should definitely be avoided.

What can be done to avoid or reduce the risk of developing cancer? It has been discovered that by adding cherries, blueberries, or vitamin E to meat will reduce the possibility of carcinogens developing. Meats also should be cooked at a low heat—no more than 200 degrees.

The head of the Research and Development Department of the Swedish National Food Administration has demonstrated that overcooking foods other than meats can be harmful also. Baking or frying some starchy foods causes the formation of acrylamide. Acrylamide causes cancer in laboratory animals.

In general, the more any food is cooked the greater the difficulty the body has in digesting and metabolizing it. This can snowball into all kinds of medical problems. Partially digested food remains in the gut, becoming toxic (poisonous). This in turn can migrate and attack an individual's weakest system. The best method to cook food is through steaming, stewing, or by using a slow crock cooker.

The closer foods are eaten in their raw state, the better the body will digest it and absorb all its nutrients. Cooked foods lose various amounts of precious vitamins and minerals.

DANGERS OF HIGH TEMPERATURE COOKING

Studies have revealed that over-cooking any food can be dangerous. The head of the Research and Development Department of the Swedish National Food Administration, Mr. Leif Busk, released a report which stated that the overcooking of some baked and fried starchy foods causes the formation of acrylamide. Acrylamide is a white, odorless cancer causing agent. It has been discovered in foods as diverse as potato chips, french fries, bread, rice, and cereal. This chemical is currently used in the treatment of sewage and waste products and in the manufacture of certain other chemicals, plastics, and dyes.

Why hasn't the public been warned about this carcinogen before now? It was never suspected that acrylamide would wind up in the food supply. The chemical's connection to food was found out somewhat by accident in 2002 by Swedish researchers. America's Food and Drug Administration (FDA), England's Food Standards Agency, and other nations' agencies have confirmed the Swedish study. It was found that acrylamide was present in significant levels when food was baked, fried, grilled, or roasted.

Acrylamide is known to cause cancer and neurotoxic effects in laboratory animals. It damages the nervous system of people who are exposed to it at work. The FDA is now investigating exactly how acrylamide will affect humans who ingest this chemical from food.

As stated in *Cooking Meats at High Temperatures*, the higher the temperature that any food is cooked, the more difficult it is for the body to digest it. The harder it is for the body to digest food, the longer it stays in the stomach. This means that the nutrients from foods on a cellular level are not being absorbed. This often leads to the body becoming poisoned.

Every food has what is known as its *heat labile point*. This is the temperature at which a food's chemical makeup is changed. Our body is programmed to digest foods at a predetermined chemical makeup. This comes from centuries of preparing and eating cooked foods. God created within our cellular structure the ability to adapt to changing circumstances. God originally created man an herbivore where no cooking was required. He probably didn't begin cooking until after God allowed him to eat meat, and then only after he had discovered fire. When food is cooked past its heat labile point, our bodies do not understand the new chemical configuration.

Food remaining in the gut due to incomplete digestion becomes toxic. Carbohydrates begin to ferment, proteins start to putrefy, and fats start to become rancid. The gastrointestinal tract becomes irritated and its cells become larger. When this happens, the undigested or partially digested food gets into the blood stream, a condition known as the "leaky gut syndrome." Moving through the blood stream, the partially digested food causes many problems for the body. Known as macromolecules, the undigested or partially digested food particles can go to the head and produce allergy-like symptoms such as runny eyes, scratchy throat, sinusitis, and sneezing. If the macromolecules reach the brain, they can cause headaches, anger, fatigue, schizophrenia, and perspiration. When they hit the joints they cause arthritis. If they impact the nerves, multiple sclerosis is the result. The macromolecules will tend to affect a person's weakest point. Everyone is affected differently.

What is the solution to the multiple problems which can be caused by high temperature cooking? Do not overcook food and stay away from over-processed foods such as potato chips and french fries. The best way to cook food is by lightly steaming it, stewing it, or by using a slow crock cooker. Food eaten in its raw, natural state is best. I now eat all of my vegetables raw. In addition to what I have listed above, avoid eating fried, barbecued, pasteurized, dried and other over-cooked and over-processed food that are found in cake mixes, dried milk, dried eggs, pizza mixes, and dairy products.

MICROWAVING IS DANGEROUS

The problems caused by cooking foods in a microwave oven are in addition to those caused by cooking at high temperatures. Just what you need, right? I just told you to give up BARbecuing your favorite meats. And now you have to throw away your microwave oven. Just kidding, folks. But we will examine the problems caused by cooking in a microwave oven. Note the following issues:

The Journal of the Science of Food and Agriculture found that:

Broccoli which was cooked in a microwave oven in some water lost up to 97% of its necessary antioxidants. Streamed broccoli lost only 11%!

Microwaving causes carcinogenic substances from plastic and paper plates or covers to mix with the food.

A woman who had received a blood transfusion died

because the blood she had been given was warmed up in a microwave oven. Warming blood is routine and safe by methods other than microwaving.

Microwaving causes vitamin B12 to be broken down into inactive and ineffective components.

Microwave ovens heat food by causing it to resonate at very high frequencies. This process causes the chemical structure of the food to change. This change is harmful and never beneficial. It has the potential of leading to health problems. It is well documented that microwave ovens produce carcinogens in milk and cereal products. It also reduces the body's ability to assimilate B-complex and Vitamins C and E and important minerals.

A little history on microwave ovens will prove enlightening. Believe it or not but the Nazis are credited with inventing the microwave oven. They used them for massive meal preparation during the invasion of Russia. After World War II, the Russians studied the biological effects of these ovens. The results of their investigations so alarmed the Russians that they outlawed microwave ovens in 1976! This should tell you something. This information has been suppressed and intentionally overlooked in this country. That should tell you something too!

I should have had this section in Chapter 2. The only difference is that Chapter 2 dealt with technological improvements which resulted in decreased physical activity. The appearance of microwave ovens in consumer homes results in a dangerous decline in physical *health*.

Growing up the 50s and 60s meant eating food cooked in a traditional oven. Microwave ovens did not exist in the homes back then. Thank God! But now that they are here, I was caught up in the ease of use and fast cooking and reheating times just as you are now. Because the information which I have just shared with you is not widely publicized, I was not aware of the dangers microwaving causes.

The truth is almost overwhelming. There has been an alarming increase of health issues stemming from poor nutrition and lack of physical exercise. And now we have this issue. Technology carries a curse as well as a blessing. The issue with the unnatural microwaving of foods, however, is something I cannot ignore. When it comes to a decision between my health and concern with the time issue, the time issue goes the way of the dinosaur. My health takes precedence. I no longer use the oven.

I recently purchased the DVD set *Star Trek- The Original Series* (Volume 2). This set encompassed the 1967—1968 season. One particular episode had a star ship captain thinking he had found the "fountain of youth" on another planet. It turns out that he was mistaken. Ship's surgeon Dr. Leonard McCoy, known as "Bones" by Captain James Kirk, said that he could do what the mythological fountain of youth was thought to have been able to accomplish with a *good diet and exercise*. I found that very interesting. It was known back in the 60s that there was no magic pill for longevity. A good diet and exercise is still the answer in this 21st century.

The typical American diet is high in saturated fat and cholesterol which are derived from meat, diary products, and eggs. Cholesterol is found only in animal products (meat) whereas saturated fat is found in animal and dairy products. Diets high in saturated fat promote obesity.

Have you noticed the many television commercials by Big Pharma promoting their cholesterol lowering drugs? The reason why the pharmaceutical industry is saturating the commercial cable stations with these advertisements is because they have a huge investment in cholesterol lowering drugs. They are their biggest sellers. Right now approximately 12 million people are on these particular drugs. This amounts to billions of dollars in annual sales. The industry downplays the importance of proper nutrition and exercise in controlling high cholesterol. God forbid someone finds that he can control his cholesterol levels without drugs!

Even though heredity could be a factor in high cholesterol

levels, these cholesterol lowering drugs are not the answer. All the person who is concerned about his cholesterol has to do is implement a healthy diet and exercise program. Of course this means a significant loss of profit for Big Pharma. They will do anything to prevent that from happening.

GOD'S CANCER CURE

We are being told that there is an ongoing battle to find the cause and cure for cancer. Is this reality? Do drug manufacturers really want to find a cure for cancer? A cure will render their current crop of chemotherapy and other cancer-fighting drugs unnecessary. Keep in mind that there is a difference between "treating" and "curing." Drugs manufactured to "treat" symptoms are guaranteed to have an ever-growing and permanent market. Any drug that cures a disease will find its market shrinking as more and more patients recover. A growing market equates to growing profits; a shrinking market directly equates to shrinking profits. You tell me if Big Pharma is really trying to find a cure.

> "For the love of money is the root of all evil: which while some have coveted after, they have erred from the faith, and pierced themselves through with many sorrows" (I Timothy 6:10).

Every drug on the market, whether prescription or nonprescription, *treats* the symptoms of medical problems. This means that every synthetic drug manufactured by Big Pharma just masks the results or symptoms of the problem. When just the symptoms of a disease are treated, the patient becomes a life long customer. This is what Big Pharma wants. But, if you find the cause of the symptom, and address that cause, the patient will be symptom free. Doesn't that sound reasonable to you? It's obvious why Big Pharma isn't concerned with finding the cause of disease. They would put themselves out of business. What CEO in his right mind is willing to let billions of dollars in sales go by the wayside?

As publicly traded companies, the pharmaceutical industry has a responsibility to its shareholders. They *have* to make money.

But here is something Big Pharma doesn't want you to know. You *don't* need them. I can say that from personal experience. I have *never* had to take prescription or nonprescription drugs. Cancer can be prevented. And even if contracted, Big Pharma's synthetic drugs aren't the answer. These drugs are responsible for causing other problems as time progresses which themselves will require other expensive medication. This sets up what is known as the *domino effect*. You are prescribed drug A for high blood pressure. In time some other condition arises which is a result of faithfully taking drug A. So now your doctor prescribes drug B for the symptoms which are the result of drug A. And on it goes, so on and so forth. The drugs are also responsible for patient deaths (remember Vioxx?) and harmful side effects.

Research has shown that over 1/3 of the 7 million cancer deaths in 2001 were due to lifestyle and environmental factors. Unlike the environment, we can control our lifestyle. Cancer prevention will require a *change* in lifestyle. That however is a small price to pay compared to the alternative. Diet is the first thing which must be altered. In line with the Word of God, and His directive to Adam, the bulk of food intake should be from plant sources. 5 to 13 servings of fruit and vegetables should be eaten daily. Other plant sources such as whole grains (wheat, bran) and legumes (beans, peas, and lentils) should also be consumed. All food sources should be organic. These foods will provide you with plenty of fiber. The typical diet should include 25 to 35 grams of fiber daily. Do the best you can. Non-organic fruit and vegetables as well as legumes are saturated with cancer causing insecticides and pesticides.

I should clarify what I mean by "diet." "Diet" doesn't mean starvation. A healthy diet means eating on a regular basis. I am using the word in the sense of what should be eaten. Ideally, one's diet should consist of 5 or 6 small, nutritious meals spaced evenly throughout the day. I want to emphasize 'small.' Portion control is a must. You should include a source of protein in each meal. This becomes even more important if you are on a weight-loss program. You should cut back on your carb intake but maintain adequate protein to keep from losing your lean muscle mass.

There are good fats which you should include in the diet. Omega 3 fatty acids and monounsaturated fats should form the majority of the fats that you consume. One of the reasons why the Mediterranean diet is so successful is that it includes a lot of monounsaturated fat such as that found in olive oil (make sure it is *extra virgin*). Canola oil is also a good source of monounsaturated oil. Cancer is not prevalent in Eskimos who eat huge quantities of fat. Their fat however comes in the form of Omega 3 fatty acids from all the seafood they eat. Red meat should be eaten only occasionally. It is high in saturated fat, and if non-organic, may be pumped full of hormones and steroids. Eat only the leanest cuts of red meat. Preferable to red meat are chicken and turkey breasts, and fish. A study undertaken in 1998 showed that men who ate less animal fat (red meat) and more vegetable fat (monounsaturated) had a lower incidence of prostate cancer. One thing researchers have realized is that obese men have a higher rate of prostate cancer while obese women have a higher rate of breast cancer. A healthy weight needs to be maintained through diet and exercise. There is just no getting around it.

Because of the issue of hormones, pasteurization, and homogenization, I would avoid drinking cow's milk. Do as I did. Substitute heart healthy soy milk (the brand I use is Silk). Of course hydrogenated and partially hydrogenated fats (trans fatty acids) should be avoided entirely. I used to eat veggie burgers until I realized that they were full of chemical additives (which I discuss in Chapter 4). They are also processed. I no longer include them in my diet.

Meats preserved with nitrite should be eliminated entirely from the diet. This can include hot dogs, ham, and sandwich meats such as salami and bologna. All processed foods should be avoided.

Begin an exercise program. It doesn't matter what type of exercise you do, just do it consistently. You should exercise at least three days per week. Whatever exercise you choose should elevate the heart rate. For older adults who want an exercise which applies the least amount of stress on the knees, I would suggest walking.

You, yes *you*, can join me in living a *quality* life. What is a "quality" life? It's that abundant life that Jesus came to give you. It's a life where you are able to concentrate on and apply all of your energies into your career and ministry for the Lord. It's a life where you won't be distracted by aches and pains—or by financial worries due to ever increasing prescription costs—or by a body constantly getting sick. Don't sit there and rationalize that it's supposed to be that way. Getting older doesn't mean that you have to *age*. We are all getting older. Your five year old child is getting *older*. But you *don't* have to age.

I reject the notion that just because I am in my 50s that I should be experiencing arthritis, high blood pressure, joint pain, or any other affliction commonly attributed to "old age." I am not suggesting that you abandon common sense. I am not going to attempt to work out in the manner and with the poundage that I did thirty years ago. But I still work out hard and consistently. Don't make yourself a prisoner of negative thoughts. Remember Proverbs 23:7a. "For as he thinketh in his heart, so is he. . . " I know that according to the Word of God I don't have to accept the devil's lie.

One thing that God *won't* do is force anyone to fully experience the abundant life. He made it possible but we must make the decision to respond. After Peter preached on the day of Pentecost, the Jews responded by asking, ". . . Men and brethren, what shall we do?" (Acts 2:37b). We have to make the conscious decision to make a drastic change in lifestyle—a decision *to do*. Once that is done, many of the physical problems that you have been praying about will disappear. This is something under *your* control. Don't think that God is just going to give you a healthy body weight in order to rid you of your medical problem. It would be a different matter if the medical condition was beyond your control. Then you would ask the elders of your church to pray for healing.

There is a saying which goes like this: *for things to change, I must change.* Paul told the Roman Christians that they had to be transformed by the renewing of their minds (Romans 12:2). The mind must be transformed from one of helpless resignation of the status quo (quietly accepting your condition), to trashing the status quo and renewing the mind with life changing thoughts. Just because things have always been a certain way doesn't mean that they have to continue that same way!

In the introduction to this book I said that God has several universal principles operating in this world. These principles will benefit anyone—saved or unsaved. Build your physical life around exercise and good nutrition and you *will* reap the rewards. Disregard these things and I guarantee you a "not so abundant" life. As a matter of fact, I guarantee that your life will be downright miserable.

DOCTORS AND NUTRITION

Let me begin this section by saying that I have no grudge against doctors. I don't disrespect them nor do I dislike them. They perform a valuable service to our society. After all, Luke, after whom the New Testament book was named, was a physician. Even Jesus realized that doctors provide a value and a service to the community. I also respect the fact that doctors undergo many years of training even after their undergraduate degree program.

Having said that, let me now state that doctors, for all their studying and training, *do not know everything* concerning the body and the various diseases and illnesses which attack it. Doctors are not gods. Why am I bringing up the subject? I'm glad you asked. There seems to be a general attitude that doctors have the answer to any and every question a patient, or potential patient, can ask of them. People seem to think that doctors know everything. I had that same perception myself at one time. I sense this yet while listening and talking to people. There is only one who knows everything about everything—*God*.

The perception of unlimited knowledge is not the doctor's fault. The general public has put them on a pedestal and now looks to doctors as "all knowing." The consensus is that their knowledge is boundless. But doctors are only human. They are subject to the same limitations and biases as any other person in any other profession, or skill. There was a time when doctors did not know the dangers of cigarette smoking. Not only did some of them smoke, but they recommended it to others. This was not done out of maliciousness, neither were they on Big Tobacco's payroll. *They just didn't know!*

A few months ago I purchased a book called *The Powerfood Nutrition Plan* written by Susan M. Kleiner. She states in this book that before she focused on becoming a nutritionist, she very much wanted to go to a medical school. She found out something through that process which astounded her.

> ... So after taking the exam to get into medical school, I went to speak with the dean of admissions at Case Western Reserve University School of Medicine, who was the father of a good friend of mine. He knew me well, and I had a long talk, and he said, "Susan, I'd love to have you in our medical school, but the fact is that you would go through 4 years and not learn anything about what you're interested in: health. *We teach people how to treat disease. . .*"[54]

Did you get that? Doctors are *only* taught how to *treat* disease and *prescribe* medication. By the way, no doctor can *heal* anyone. That is the prerogative of God and God alone. Why do I bring this up? Well, when it comes to the basis for a patient's cancer or high cholesterol or diabetes or heart disease or asthma, or the many other medical conditions resulting from lifestyle choices, doctors are not trained to recognize these symptoms as stemming from poor nutrition and/or a lack of exercise. In other words, doctors are not trained by medical schools to look for the *cause* of the symptom. They are only trained to treat the symptoms with medication. The underlying problem goes undetected and the patient is condemned to a lifetime of prescription drugs. As an example, high blood pressure is treated by a doctor giving a prescription for high blood pressure medication. He may also provide the patient with a diet to go along with the medication. But he would *never* give a diet plan *without* the medication! The doctor has not been trained to look for the high blood pressure as being a consequence of poor nutrition. If he were so trained, he would recommend better nutrition, and write out what that nutrition plan would consist of. Prescription drugs would not be on the agenda.

Doctors are also heavily courted by salespersons from Big Pharma. These salespersons demonstrate their particular medications, and give out samples. There are many incentives given to doctors for 'pushing' certain prescription drugs. This is just the reality of the situation. ". . .From their first rounds as residents, doctors travel in a world increasingly dominated by drug company salespeople proffering meals, office supplies, entertainment and even cash to speak at conferences or sit on advisory boards. . . Some physicians have been paid lucrative consulting retainers for no specific work; others are paid to put their names on articles ghostwritten by industry employees. . . "[55]

To say that there is a conflict of interest between doctors and their patients and Big Pharma is an understatement. And as always, it's the patients who get the short end of the stick. Not only may there be cheaper generic drugs available, but the doctor, if so inclined, will not seek alternate natural products (natural herbs and cures from God). As Chris Rock said in his hilarious movie *Head of State* a few years back, "that ain't right."

There are 125 medical schools in this country. Of this number, only 24% have a mandatory course in nutrition. And out of his four years of medical school, the average doctor receives only *about three hours* of nutrition training! You obviously don't want a physician making a life and death decision on a medical problem which comes from eating a highly refined, nutrient deficit diet. He's not trained for that. What to do? Get not only second and third opinions, but also seek out alternate (natural) methods. This applies to everything with the exception of that which doctors are really qualified for—physical injuries and the like. Doctors are totally unqualified to answer detailed nutrition related questions. For that a qualified nutritionist should be sought.

When it comes to the beneficial effects of supplements, herbs, or any of the other natural remedies for the body, doctors have no clue. Their answers to any nutrition questions will be based solely on the possible negative effect any natural supplement or herb will have on you when it comes into contact with the medication. They will question the natural supplement of course, and insist that you not take it. But they have been programmed to believe that the medication itself is beneficial.

I am not maligning doctors and saying that they all have ulterior motives. Most of them are acting solely on their training, and most are truly concerned with you, the patient. But there are a few rotten, money hungry apples which spoil the entire barrel.

EAT ONLY ORGANIC

In order to eat food that is as close to nature as possible, you have to sacrifice and buy organic. I am talking about meats, fruits, vegetables, cereal—everything. Modern food processing leaves the public no choice. Not only does the American public have to contend with meat and dairy products contaminated with growth hormones and antibiotics, and having dead animals as part of their diet, the animals to be slaughtered are also crammed together in filth and squalor. The constant exposure to this filthy and unsanitary environment breeds disease. To combat this disease, the animals are given antibiotics. Residual amounts of herbicides, hormones, and antibiotics remain in the animal's tissue after they are slaughtered. This means that they find their way to your dinner plate.

An interesting study revealed that if a child is placed on a total organic food program, all traces of herbicides will vanish in only five days. These contaminants accumulate in human fatty tissue and build up over time. Hormones can cause gender confusion, obesity, and multi-generational cancer; pesticides are carcinogenic (cancer causing); hydrogenated fats (trans fats) have been linked to heart disease, cancer, diabetes, and obesity. Genetically modified foods can cause IBS (irritable bowel syndrome), Crohn's disease, and autism. The antibiotics that remain in slaughtered meat will compromise your immune system. In addition to the hormones and antibiotics, the government allows food companies to put thousands of artificial chemical additives in non organic food. These additives are included to prolong shelf life, increase sweetness or saltiness, and improve appearance and taste.

When man attempts to change or improve or make larger anything in nature, he is approaching the forbidden zone of God's domain. He is in effect playing God. Remember the story of Frankenstein? Doctor Frankenstein went beyond the ethical boundaries of medical science in attempting to bring life from dead human carcasses. The result was something the doctor could not have predicted. Consequently he was destroyed by his own creation. The same is true with genetic modification. Science is playing in uncharted waters and we the consumers are going to pay the price. Tampering in areas which are forbidden to man reminds me of Proverbs 11:29a. "He that troubleth his own house shall inherit the wind. . . " These are prophetic words because we are now inheriting the wind. We are seeing the physical manifestations of genetic modifications, new chemical compounds placed in foods, and chemically stripping nutrients from whole foods. Different forms of cancers are on the rise and obesity, along with its deadly consequences, is increasing among our youth.

> . . . If you recently ate soya sauce in a Chinese restaurant, munched popcorn in a movie theatre, or indulged in an occasional candy bar—you've undoubtedly ingested this new type of food. You may have, at the time, known exactly how much salt, fat and carbohydrates were in each of these foods because regulations mandates their labeling for dietary purposes. But you would not know if the bulk of these foods, and literally every cell had been genetically altered![56]

But what exactly is genetic modification? Genetic modification involves adding new genes from some other living organism. Genes are strings of chemicals which comprise DNA. If, for instance, resistance to a pesticide is desired, the food would be genetically modified. The goal is to give new characteristics to a food that didn't have it by nature. This is truly man circumventing

God's plan with human engineering. Whereas nutritional labeling is mandatory for all foods, the government doesn't require that the food companies label that their product has been genetically modified.

CHAPTER 6:

Legal Unnatural Drugs

INTRODUCTION

Turn to any network commercial television channel and you are guaranteed to see at least one advertisement for a synthetic drug during a commercial break. Big Pharma's (the drug industry) advertising budget literally runs into the billions of dollars. These dollars are well spent on slick, Madison Avenue commercials which enthrall you in its message. They are hard to resist. These commercials are so well produced that they seem 100 percent honest. They will have you believing that only they provide the answer for your medical problem.

> ... The general public has been brainwashed by TV ads, the news media, and the FDA into believing that prescription drugs enrich their lives. Many also still believe that government agencies such as the FDA ensure that these drugs are safe and perform the way the pharmaceutical companies claim they do. Hogwash... [57]

The above quote was taken from an article entitled *Legal Drugs*

Kill, Too. This article also mentioned the now infamous drug Vioxx. Vioxx was on the market for five years. It has been estimated that between 88,000 and 139,000 heart attacks and strokes were related to the drug's use. Big Pharma is not your friend; neither is the FDA.

> "... The public seems to genuinely believe that drugs advertised on TV are safe, in spite of the plethora of side effects listed by the commercial's narrator, ranging from diarrhea to death... Remember all those TV ads heralding the wonders of Vioxx?... "[58]

Human nature being what it is, the very drugs consumers see advertised over and over again on TV are the ones they ask their doctors for. That's why TV commercials are so important for the drug industry. Big Pharma has very deep pockets to promote their prescription and nonprescription drugs. The consumer, despite the required disclaimer of possible side effects, feels that these drugs must be safe. After all, if they were dangerous, the government wouldn't allow them to be advertised. The tragedy with Vioxx should be a wake up call to all of us. Safety of the consumer is not Big Pharma's or the FDA's major concern. Profits are their one and only concern.

All drugs advertised by the pharmaceutical industry are synthetic and have been sanctioned by the Federal Drug Administration (FDA). This is why I refer to them as 'legal' *unnatural* drugs. They are unnatural because they are chemical compounds formulated in a laboratory and are not 'recognized' by the body. This is why they cause the side effects that the pharmaceutical companies have to announce. But what they don't tell you is that these drugs could lead to far greater medical risks.

Also these legal unnatural drugs are not formulated to 'cure' anyone of anything. They are manufactured to simply mask and relieve the symptom of the real cause of the medical problem. For instance, cancer is a symptom of an underlying problem. That problem could be toxic buildup in body tissues, too much saturated fat, a diet high in refined carbohydrates or processed foods, or any number of other things.

VIOXX, IT'S ALL ABOUT MONEY

Kevin Trudeau repeats over and over in his book *Natural Cures "They" Don't Want You To Know About* that, "...It's all about the money..." He is absolutely right. When it comes to the pharmaceutical industry, enormous profits are at stake. For anyone to think that the pharmaceutical industry is willingly going to give up billions of dollars for the sake of ethics or morality indicates that person still believes in the tooth fairy. "For the love of money is the root of all evil..." (I Timothy 6:10a).

There were two rival pharmaceutical companies, Merck and Pfizer, who were both working on medications for arthritis pain. Merck's arthritis pain drug is called Vioxx and Pfizer's arthritis pain drug is called Celebrex. You've heard of both of them. Which pharmaceutical company would finish their product, test it, submit it for FDA approval, and upon approval, market it, first? Keep in mind that billions of dollars are involved.

Merck, not willing to have rival Pfizer place its product on the market first, rushed Vioxx to market despite evidence that it was the cause of cardiovascular problems. MSNBC says, "...Like jurors in five Vioxx-related trials before it, the jury saw dozens of emails, internal Merck documents and safety study reports and heard testimony from a parade of cardiology experts, academics and Merck executives..."[59] Merck was aware of clinical studies which suggested that Vioxx was causing heart attacks and strokes. The pharmaceutical company went so far as to petition the FDA to tone down a new warning label in April of 2002. All this time anywhere from 88,000 to 139,000 heart attacks and strokes were a direct result of the use of Vioxx.

When a publicly traded company is attempting to beat a competitor to market, it doesn't have time for comprehensive testing—a process which could, and in the case of a product to be used for human consumption, should take years. *It's all about the money*. People are a secondary consideration. Merck proved that, and that fact came out in court.

John McDarby, the 77 year old plaintiff in a Vioxx lawsuit who won a judgment for $4.5 million in compensatory damages, racked up another victory. John had taken Vioxx for four years before he suffered a heart attack which resulted in a broken hip from a fall related to the attack. John was recently awarded $9 million in punitive damages for a grand total of $13.5 million. The jurors trying the case said that Merck 'dragged its feet' in notifying its customers of the heart attack and stroke risks, and in taking its time in changing Vioxx's product label. The punitive damage accuses Merck of "bad conduct." According to New Jersey law, this case could be referred to the county prosecutor and the state's Attorney General's office to determine if a criminal act was perpetrated.

It's all about the money. Big Pharma is goal oriented. That goal is to make as much profit as it possibly can. It cares nothing for those whose lives were destroyed through heart attacks and strokes related to the use of Vioxx. And it cares nothing for the families who lost loved ones from having taken Vioxx.

What does Vioxx and Celebrex and the hundreds of other drugs produced by the pharmaceutical industry have to do with *living a God-glorifying life through good health*? The point that I am trying to stress is that God doesn't want His people to be enslaved by synthetic drugs. What makes this all the more sad is that the drug makers have no conscience and are therefore opposed to the love of God. To rely on health destroying synthetic drugs helps to support Satan's kingdom.

Neither the pharmaceutical industry nor the food industry are forthcoming about the validity of the many conclusive studies to show that their products can lead to cancer, multiple sclerosis, heart disease, asthma, high blood pressure, and many other deadly health issues. They have too much to lose. They are no different than Big Tobacco. These big money interests will lie, deceive, and confuse the issue to keep their loyal customers, loyal. I am not tarring the ordinary worker at these industries with the same brush by any means. Most of them are honest and just doing their jobs to support their families. I am talking about executive management who is responsible for the bottom line—the greedy money-grubbers who would do anything to make a profit. *It's all about the money*!

TYPE 2 DIABETES

This disease used to be known as *adult-onset diabetes*. At one time this affliction was confined to the adult population. Now children are being diagnosed with type 2 diabetes. The causes of type 2 diabetes are, among other things, obesity, a high sugar diet, sedentary life, etc. There is now a body of research that indicates that the current crop of drugs used to treat type 2 diabetes raises the risk of dying from cardiovascular disease.

Type 2 diabetes provides a gold mine for the pharmaceutical industry. The statistics are a cause for concern. Consider the following: 1) 18 million Americans have type 2 diabetes 2) over 1/3 of new cases reported occur in children and teenagers and 3) the total cost of type 2 diabetes is estimated at 132 billion dollars in the United States alone!

Contrary to what the pharmaceutical industry says, a change in lifestyle is the *only* way to combat this disease. It is certainly the safest. Big Pharma is only interested in *treating* this moneymaker, certainly not to prevent it or cure it. They will tell you that diet and exercise matters, but, their drug must also be used. They are not so stupid as to cause any decline in usage of their big money-making drugs.

Most of the drugs used to treat type 2 diabetes belong to a group known as sulfonylureas. "... Sulfonylurea drugs stimulate the beta cells of the pancreas to squeeze out more insulin. This same mechanism constricts arteries, increases blood pressure, and reduces blood flow to the heart—which can result in chest pain and sudden death..."[60] In 2001 the number of prescriptions for these type 2 diabetes drugs was over 32.5 million. It has been discovered that these drugs also seem to increase the risk of dying from cancer.

Big Pharma Is Disease Mongering

Are there no limits to the depths to which the pharmaceutical industry will sink in order to increase its profits? It seems not. They are not satisfied with taking in more than three times the average profits of other fortune 500 companies. *They want more.* The *British Medical Journal* presented an article entitled 'Selling Sickness: The Pharmaceutical Industry and Disease Mongering.' Their investigation found out that Big Pharma has begun focusing on common symptoms and calling it a disease so that a prescription can be given for it. This has the intended effect of enveloping more potential customers which of course means more money in Big Pharma's coffers.

It's interesting that an English publication broke the story about "disease mongering" and not some American medical publication. It's interesting but not unusual. You see, England has laws on the books against their pharmaceutical companies engaging in 'disease mongering.' America has no such laws.

So concerned is Big Pharma with increasing their consumer base, that they spend more dollars on marketing than they do on research and development. If that fact doesn't wake you up to the reality that the pharmaceutical industry's interests are on profits, and profits alone, nothing will. So the fact that they are willing to stoop to such practices as *disease mongering* doesn't come as a surprise to me. "... The practice of 'disease mongering' by the drug industry is promoting non-existent illnesses or exaggerating minor ones for the sake of profits..."[61] This article gives examples such as female sexual dysfunction, attention deficit hyperactivity disorder (ADHD), and restless leg syndrome. I have seen drugs for restless leg syndrome advertised on television. As if that weren't enough, pharmaceutical companies are also throwing the symptoms of menopause into the mix.

This dastardly practice will create thousands more prescription drug addicts, and bring in millions more dollars into the overflowing coffers of Big Pharma. "... A lot of money can be made from healthy people who believe they are sick..."[62] New cholesterol guidelines provide a good example of increasing a consumer base. The number of new people taking prescription drugs such as Lipitor, Zocor, Prevachol, Lescol, Mevacor, and Crestor will jump tremendously. This translates into a nearly three-fold increase of cholesterol lowering drug usage.

I believe that the public should be aware of such practices. They look upon the pharmaceutical companies and doctors as knowing all there is to know about disease and their treatment. They are also looked upon as having the public's welfare at heart. The last thing the public suspects from Big Pharma is ulterior motives and hidden agendas.

Unfortunately, with today's "get rich quick" or 'cure me with a pill' mentality, the public is easy prey for slick advertising and trusted doctors dispensing prescriptions as though they were candy. Today's overfed and undernourished society would rather 'pop' a prescription or over-the-counter pill instead of making a lifestyle change which would allow the body to heal itself naturally. And it's also unfortunate that we can do everything under the sun with the exception of taking care of *the temple of the Holy Ghost* through exercise.

The *Sunday Star-Ledger* carried an article on the front page named 'An America on the go also is on the grow.' "Even the test dummies are putting on weight. As Americans get heavier, the people who build and regulate cars, boats and planes are trying to keep up, adjusting design standards and safety rules to account for newly recognized safety risks posed by those extra pounds per person. . . " (April 30, 2006).

The article went on to mention that the Centers for Disease Control (CDC) say that 65% of Americans are overweight. Statistics show that from 1960 to 2002 the average man's weight went from 166 pounds to 191 pounds; the average woman's weight grew from 140 to 164 pounds. This is an alarming increase. The culprit for this increase in weight and accompanying girth are empty and nutritionally deficient calories. This epidemic of overweight and obese Americans has a direct bearing on automobile safety. Studies have shown that the more overweight a person is, the more likely that person is liable to die in a crash.

There is also a direct correspondence between pounds gained

and the medical symptoms that crop up. As these medical symptoms such as hypertension, diabetes, cancer, etc. appear, synthetic drugs are prescribed. As these drugs are taken, side effects may manifest themselves, and they may cause other, far greater problems in the future. No doubt when that occurs, other drugs will be prescribed to alleviate those symptoms. And so the vicious cycle continues to spin.

DRUG STORES, DRUG STORES EVERYWHERE

When we baby-boomers (those born between 1946 and 1964) were growing up, our neighborhoods had the popular corner drug store. That was the only place where you could get prescriptions filled, or buy aspirin. Back in the late 50s and early 60s, our corner drug store was located at the corner of Harrison and Monticello Avenues in Jersey City, New Jersey. That was right down the street from our family which lived at 45 Harrison Avenue. These drug stores were 'mom and pop' type businesses. The drug chains that we are so familiar with today did not exist back then.

Today, drug stores or pharmacies have multiplied like rabbits. This is a sad commentary on our society. Why? Well for one thing it shows in great detail how our dependency on prescription and nonprescription drugs has grown. When I was growing up, the corner drug store was adequate to dispense all the pharmaceuticals the neighborhood ever needed. Today it seems as though drugs have become another food group. They have become staples.

Drug chains such as Eckerd, cvs, and Walgreens have multiple stores just in one town. And as if that weren't bad enough, supermarket chains such as ShopRite, PathMark and Stop&Shop have pharmacies inside them. This says volumes about today's legal unnatural drug culture. Not only has the number of patients increased, but these same patients are taking multiple prescriptions.

PHARMACEUTICAL DRUGS
ARE NOT THE ANSWER

"... Over 750,000 people actually do die in the United States every year... they die from something far more common and rarely perceived by the public as dangerous: modern medicine... "[63]

Hard to believe, isn't it? We think of hospitals as sanctuaries of life and doctors as miracle men who can do no wrong. And what about prescription drugs? We think of them as a panacea for whatever ails us. I am not implying that hospitals are bad or that physicians are witch doctors in white smocks. But take a peek behind the veneer. You might be surprised.

In 2003 doctors Gary Null, Carolyn Dean, Martin Feldman, Debora Rasio, and Dorothy Smith released a medical report they titled *Death by Medicine*. This report proves that the number one cause of death in America is not heart disease or lung cancer, but is a result of the medical profession. The number of deaths due to heart disease in 2001 was 699,697; the number of deaths in 2001 from cancer was 553,251. The total number of deaths in America in 2001 which were medical in origin was 783,936! Of this number, 106,000 deaths were the result of adverse drug reactions. You can imagine the number of patients who suffered some other medical issue, whether temporary or permanent, but survived. Medical error accounted for 98,000 deaths while unnecessary procedures accounted for 37,136. The annual price tag for iatrogenic deaths (deaths from medical causes) is $282 billion. This figure is not only astounding, but conservative. Not all iatrogenic deaths are reported. Some estimate that the dollar figure could conceivably be twenty times higher!

... Medicine is not taking into consideration the following monumentally important aspects of a healthy human organism: (a) stress and how it adversely affects the immune system and life processes; (b) *insufficient exercise*; (c) *excessive caloric intake*; (d) *highly-processed and denatured foods grown in denatured and chemically-damaged soil*; and (e) exposure to tens of thousands of environmental toxins. Instead of minimizing these disease-causing factors, we actually cause more illness through medical technology, diagnostic testing, over-use of medical and surgical procedures, *and overuse of pharmaceutical drugs*. The huge disservice of this therapeutic strategy is the result of little effort or money being appropriated for preventing disease. . . [64]

I highlighted *insufficient exercise, excessive caloric intake, highly-processed and denatured foods grown in denatured and chemically damaged soil* in the above quote because I specifically address these issues in this book. Take a look at reason (b), *insufficient exercise*. This explanation assumes some form of exercise. Many people get no exercise *at all*!

America's 'tab' for healthcare in 2004 reached $1.4 trillion. Obviously there's something very wrong here. America's health care system and its health in general should be the best in the world judging by the sheer amount of money spent. But it isn't. Our health care system is a total failure. ". . . Since Americans spend so much money on health care, they should be getting a high quality of care, right? Unfortunately, that's not the case. . . " (www.newstarget.com/009278.html.) As a matter of fact, it shouldn't be referred to as the healthcare system, but rather the *sickness* system. Not only are the numbers escalating, but our system is focusing on the wrong thing. Today's health system focuses on *treatment* when the emphasis should be on *prevention*.

> Currently, about 95% of health care dollars in the United States are spent on treating diseases, with relatively little attention paid to preventing diseases, which should be a national priority. . . (former U.S. Surgeon General David Satcher, MD, PHD.)

It's not hard to see why maintaining the status quo would be much more lucrative than by focusing on preventive care. By treating symptoms the pharmaceutical companies, doctors, and hospitals are guaranteed ever increasing income streams. If, God forbid, the health care system would put all their collective energies into *preventive maintenance*, not only would earnings decrease, but eventually some or all of the pharmaceutical companies would actually go out of business. I often tell people that if every American was like me, every pharmaceutical company would have to close its door, and hospitals' workloads would lighten substantially.

Today's *Star-Ledger* (Thursday, May 18, 2006) contained an article entitled *A spiritual life ends just shy of 110 years*. It was the story of Bertha Lee Jones who died just 2 months and 2 days before she would have celebrated her 110th birthday. Jennifer Sills, Director of Activities of the Good Shepherd Nursing Home in Hackettstown, NJ, said of Bertha, "Up to a month ago, you could sit and talk to Bertha about anything..." What is even more remarkable about Bertha Jones other than her longevity is the fact that she *was not on any prescription drug*. It is unfortunate that our society thinks that senior citizen and prescription drugs are synonymous. I can't prove what I am about to say with undisputable scientific fact, but I believe that a contributing factor to Bertha's long life was that *she did not take any prescription drugs*!

Many over-the-counter (OTC) drugs are so ubiquitous that millions of people don't think twice about taking them. Their longevity has made them seemingly innocuous. Take Tylenol for instance. Tylenol is a drug usually taken for pain relief and to reduce fever. It is commonly used for headaches, muscle aches, arthritis, colds, backaches, and toothaches. But did you know that Tylenol is the second leading cause of liver transplants?

SWEETHEARTS: THE FDA AND BIG PHARMA

> ... Adverse drug reactions are the fourth leading cause of death in America. Reactions to prescription and over-the-counter medications kill far more people annually than all illegal drug use combined.[65]

Annually, drug companies spend billions on TV commercials and print media. They spend over $12 billion a year handing out drug samples and employing sales forces to influence doctors to promote specifically branded drugs. The drug industry employs over 1,200 lobbyists, including 40 former members of Congress. Drug companies have spent close to a billion dollars since 1998 on lobbying. In 2004, drug companies and their officials contributed at least $17 million to federal election campaigns. . ."[66]

Pretty scary, isn't it? Adverse reactions to synthetic drugs are the fourth leading cause of death in America today. And then look at the money Big Pharma has at its disposal. This money is used to buy whatever is needed in order to stay in business, or should I say power? If you haven't figured it out by now, money is power. Big Pharma has a virtual monopoly on medications and drugs. While a monopoly, it simultaneously excludes the natural vitamins, herbs, and supplements that you find in health food stores. These natural products cannot be classified as drugs according to a FDA mandate. And according to the FDA, only a drug can cure a disease. So natural products cannot claim to be able to cure or prevent a disease. So if you buy a product from a health food store and it makes a statement such as "CLA has been shown to play a vital role in reducing body fat and increasing muscle tone according to human clinical studies and laboratory testing. . ." (Product: *Tonalin* CLA; The Vitamin Shoppe), it must have the following FDA disclaimer: "These statements have not been evaluated by the Food and Drug Administration. This product is not intended to diagnose, treat, cure, or prevent any disease." This tactic tends to prejudice the consumer as he considers purchasing a product which, according to the FDA, may not live up to its claims. The consumer may therefore think the product is a 'rip-off.' Or, even worse, the disclaimer may turn the potential alternative drug seeker away from all natural and homeopathic cures. Oh by the way, Tonalin CLA is one of the supplements that I use daily.

. . . The other strategy they use is to seek to confuse

by funding research that casts suspicion on food and natural nutrients as alternatives to their highly lucrative drug-based options. Don't be fooled by their illusions: all drugs typically provide you is a symptomatic Band-Aid that will only further accelerate your path toward degeneration, allowing them to sell you even more expensive Band-Aids down the line. What you should be addressing—and what they won't address because it is not profitable—are the underlying causes of your health issues. . . [67]

The Food and Drug Administration is working on behalf of its client the pharmaceutical industry, and not you the consumer. It's all politics and big money. Safety and public welfare are nowhere on the agenda. The Texans battle cry in their war with Mexico was *remember the Alamo*. My battle cry against the FDA is *remember Vioxx*. The FDA is a government agency and we tend to think of government agencies as looking out for the public's welfare, and for thoroughly testing all drugs before they are released to the public. And most of all, we think of government agencies as being completely independent. Now you know the truth. Don't trust the FDA to tell you the complete unbiased truth about any natural or homeopathic product because they are in competition, along with their client Big Pharma, against anyone or any company who promotes alternative cures. Big Pharma and its sweetheart the FDA spend huge sums of money for advertising, and to prosecute any company or individual who attempts to market a natural or homeopathic product. These individuals and companies are then completely discredited in the media.

Dr. David Graham is intimately familiar with the FDA (Federal Drug Administration). Dr. Graham blew the whistle on the deadly drug Vioxx. He is currently Associate Director for Science and Medicine in the Office of Drug Safety within the FDA. He has been with the agency for twenty years. In an interview, Dr. Graham said the following,

". . . As currently configured, the FDA is not able to adequately protect the American public. *It's more interested in protecting the interests of industry. It views industry as its client* and the client is someone whose interest you represent. Unfortunately, that is the way the FDA is currently structured. . ."[68]

The reason that I used the title that I did for this section is given by Dr. Graham in the above quote. It doesn't take a rocket scientist to figure out that the FDA's primary and total commitment is to the pharmaceutical industry, and not to the American public.

Okay, again you're asking the question, "What does this have to do with *living A God-glorifying life through good health?*" Plenty! First of all God does not want His people to be dependent on *the arms of flesh.* This is especially true if the arms of flesh are not at all concerned about you as a person, but with *filthy lucre.* Remember what I have been saying all along? "For the love of money is the root of all evil. . . " (I Timothy 6:10a). Big Pharma's only concern is money. Billions of dollars in profits are at stake. Don't think that they are going to be conscience stricken anytime in the near future. God on the other hand has your best interests at heart. "Beloved, I wish above all things that thou mayest prosper and be in health, even as thy soul prospereth" (III John 2).

It is solely up to you to trust God at His Word. He desires for you to have a healthy and fit body. In order to get and maintain a healthy and fit body we must subscribe to God's principles. Our bodies must be nourished with wholesome food. Wholesome food means food as close to nature as possible. That means as far away from processing as possible. By eating organic fruit, vegetables, whole grains, meat if you so choose, and plenty of water, you supply your body with the raw materials it needs to build and repair. This will enable you to remain healthy and you won't need to take toxic synthetic prescription and nonprescription drugs from Big Pharma. All attempts should be made to wean ones self off these drugs.

The pharmaceutical industry has a virtual stranglehold on America. As a nation we take a disproportionate amount of prescription drugs. We have been brainwashed, deceived, hoodwinked, bamboozled, tricked, led astray, beguiled, had the wool pulled over our eyes and duped by slick television, radio, newspaper, and magazine advertising. These polished ads feature professional actors who create an aura of sincerity and trustworthiness. These shysters, Big Pharma and the ad agencies, not the professional actors, want you to believe that they sympathize with you, and that they have the products to address your health concerns. Lord have mercy. I think one of the saddest, if not the saddest, verses in the entire Bible is John 5:40. "And ye will not come to me, that ye might have life." Jesus Himself said this. I can picture Him now standing brokenhearted, tears welling up in His eyes, watching as man seeks everyone and everything but Him! Jesus, who is eternal life in the flesh, seems to be pleading with mankind to trust Him, and *only* Him. No one has to be part of the crowd which trusts Big Pharma.

Because the only voice we hear is that of Big Pharma, we tend to think that they present the only alternative to health crises. America has become overly dependent on Big Pharma. I will never become dependent on any harmful drug. America's mind set is that it is a natural progression to have to take prescription drugs as one gets older. It is deplorable that the average senior citizen has to budget hundreds of dollars a month on drugs. When a choice has to be made between buying food and drugs, and sometimes even between paying the rent and buying medication, things have gotten way out of hand. Senior citizens and all others who buy into Big Pharma's lies are being victimized.

It doesn't have to be this way. We should be victors, not victims. "Nay, in all these things we are more than conquerors through him that loved us" (Romans 8:37). You don't have to be held captive by the pharmaceutical industry. Take control of your life, your health, and your finances. Don't wait—*do it now!*

The Vioxx tragedy should have convinced you that Big Pharma is about as concerned with human life as the typical American is about Bill Gate's financial status. Tough language I know. But it shows how I feel about the situation. The pharmaceutical company Merck knew about the dangers of its drug

Vioxx but it took a whistleblower to cry out before they pulled it off the market. Don't think that those thousands of deaths directly linked to Vioxx, and others which we are not aware of, will make any difference in Big Pharma's business model because they won't. The profits are simply too great.

I am a living witness that you don't need Big Pharma. There are thousands of natural alternatives which are fighting an uphill battle to get publicized. And who is the major opposition against natural cures becoming well known and used? You guessed it, Big Pharma. God forbid that the American public should find out that there exist cures for cancer, multiple sclerosis, diabetes, high blood pressure, and dozens of other major health issues. Or God forbid that the public should find out that there are alternative treatments to chemotherapy when cancer has been diagnosed. Chemotherapy treatments and unnecessary surgeries generate thousands, no millions, of dollars for hospitals and Big Pharma. It's all about money. It's not a health issue, but rather a money issue.

If you take care of your body as God commanded you to, you will not be at the mercy of Big Pharma. Neither will you be at the mercy of some unscrupulous doctors, and hospitals which care more about money than about your welfare. If you don't, and you follow the path of least resistance, you are at their mercy. I am not the only voice crying out in the wilderness. There are literally thousands of others, including doctors who have *seen the light*. We are not in the clutches of Big Pharma. Personally, I never have been. That's why I can say categorically that you don't need them. If I were to stop exercising and eating nutritious organic food, then I would be preparing to place myself at the mercy of toxic drugs and unnecessary surgeries. Keep in mind that when you go against God's natural order, you will pay the price. Pharmaceutical drugs are synthetic and toxic to the body.

The term 'conflict of interest' is being heard a lot today. This occurs when someone in a position of trust, such as a lawyer, a politician, or an executive or director of a corporation, has competing professional or personal interests. Ten of the thirty two FDA drug advisers whose total votes favored the drugs Vioxx,

Celebrex, and Bextra had financial attachments to the pharmaceutical industry. One will naturally be favorable to the interests of the company which compensates for such consideration. What does this mean to the consumer? It means that despite the danger to the public scientific evidence may show concerning a specific drug, it is very likely to be approved. Big Pharma and the FDA are sweethearts. As long as financial favors are forthcoming, the FDA will never betray their lover, Big Pharma. And it doesn't matter how many lives may be at stake.

> ... More than half of the experts hired to advise the government on the safety and effectiveness of medicine have financial relationships with the pharmaceutical companies that will be helped or hurt by their decisions, a *USA TODAY* study found. These experts are hired to advise the Food and Drug Administration on which medicines should be approved for sale, what the warning labels should say and how studies of drugs should be designed. The experts are supposed to be independent, but *USA TODAY* found that 54% of the time, they have a direct financial interest in the drug or topic they are asked to evaluate. These conflicts include helping a pharmaceutical company develop a medicine, then serving on an FDA advisory committee that judges the drug. The conflicts typically include stock ownership, consulting fees or research grants... [69]

CHAPTER 7:

Exercise

INTRODUCTION

The more labor-saving devices technology provides to make our daily lives easier, the greater the need to exercise. The more that is done for us, the less we tend to do for ourselves. The latter statement is simplistically true. It is so obvious that I don't think a single individual would disagree with it. Chapter 2 of this book listed and elaborated on the many technological innovations that have eased our burdens down through the years. Alas, they are partially to blame for our problem too. America's chronic weight problem is continually growing (pun intended). The only solution is a comprehensive *weight management* program

Weight management encompasses weight loss, gain, or maintenance through exercise and nutrition. For the overwhelming majority of America's population which has a weight problem, weight management will consist of weight loss. Wouldn't it be wonderful if the majority of us were at a healthy weight? Before I began lifting weights, I considered myself underweight. I was at my present height of 5' 10" with a body weight of 145 to 150 pounds. While being underweight is not a headline generating situation, *it does indicate a problem*. "... Health problems associated with being underweight can include fighting off infection, osteoporosis, decreased muscle strength, trouble regulating body temperature and even increased risk of death..."[70]

There is always a right way to do something and a wrong way. Going about something the wrong way will give you unsatisfactory results, and leave you unfulfilled and frustrated. The right way to lose unwanted weight is by employing proper nutrition and an exercise program. One without the other will just not work. Unfortunately there is a lot of misleading and confusing information in the public realm concerning weight loss.

LET'S BE HONEST

Many people are less than honest in their appraisal of their weight. It's a fact that we all see ourselves differently than other people see us. If we could see ourselves as other people see us, we would likely all be shocked. I like what Alcoholics Anonymous teaches its people. They are taught to begin their testimonies with the phrase, "I'm an alcoholic." Everyone with a weight problem should face it by acknowledging it

Before any problem can be solved, it has to be admitted that there is a problem. If this step is not addressed, the unacknowledged problem will never be resolved. Neither will it magically go away. The number used to determine overall health is the body mass index (BMI). This index is based on an individual's height and weight. The BMI is universally recognized.

Underweight: BMI less than 18.5
Normal Weight: BMI from 18.5 thru 25
Overweight: BMI from 25 thru 29.9
Obese: BMI over 30
Morbidly Obese: BMI over 40

When a person is brutally honest about his health and weight and sincere about getting them under control, the prognosis is 100 percent success. However, if a person is less than honest about his weight and health, the approach to correcting the problems will be half-hearted at best, and doomed to failure in the end. His attempts at weight loss and better eating habits will be a challenge because he is not fully committed. There may be several reasons for this. Maybe he's doing it because he feels pressured by someone else or he is just trying to please someone else. In any case, these are not the right reasons to do it. Do it because not only is it the right thing to do in order to live a God-glorifying life through good health, but because *you* want to do it. You see the need. When you have finished reading this book, you should want to gain control of your health and weight. If you don't, I have failed. (Please help me out, I can't take failure).

I just came across an article over the internet which says that weight and height statistics are under reported in the United States. This is not surprising. People are rarely objective when it comes to themselves. Bonnie Taub-Dix, M.A., R.D., of the American Dietetic Association says that, ". . . self-reported heights and weights rarely match reality. . . " America's overweight and obesity rates are epidemic in scope. But with Americans reporting conservative height and weight figures, a bad situation is even worse than we thought. How much worse? A study reported in the *Journal of the Royal Society of Medicine* showed that for the year 2002, 29% of men were obese as opposed to the reported figure of 16%; the revised figure for women was 35% as opposed to 22%. There is a large disparity between the reported figures and those that are based in reality.

You are familiar with the old saying, *honesty is the best policy*. Well, it may be old, but it's still relevant today. It is said that confession is good for the soul. If you are part of the overweight or obese epidemic, admit it. Or as they say in ordinary street language, 'fess up. If you did admit it, good for you. It took a lot of courage. Now, don't you feel better? Sure you do. So let's get on with the business at hand of rectifying the problem.

WHAT'S MY MOTIVATION?

It's one thing to begin an exercise program. It's something

else entirely to do it day in and day out. Consistency separates the men from the boys and the women from the girls. You may ask me what kept me in the gym for 28 years. I can sum it up in one word. And that word is *discipline*. Yes, it was the D word that kept me focused.

Medical studies have shown that overweight or obese people have a shortened life span. Obesity affects others too. For instance, the infant mortality rate for babies born to obese mothers is substantially higher than for infants born to mothers of normal weight. Obese teenagers on average can expect to live 15 years shorter than a teenager of normal weight. "... The obese, and to a lesser but still significant extent the overweight, have higher rates of heart disease, diabetes, liver disorders, gallbladder disease, cancer, arthritis, and virtually every other degenerative disease..."[71]

The fact that obesity can lead to such deadly diseases as cancer and liver disorders should provide the necessary incentive to consider an exercise program. An additional reason is family. If you are a parent you want to be able to live in good health for your children, and for your grandchildren. This is especially true if your children are small. These are all good motivational factors. My father was 53 years old when I was born. His health was so good that he was able to work and provide for myself and an additional nine siblings!

Another factor is completely self-centered (I mean that in a positive way). Think of being able to wear whatever type of clothing without ever having to be self-conscious about it. Imagine the feeling of looking in the mirror and loving what you see looking back. You'll never have to be ashamed about yourself. Neither will you have to wear bulky clothing in an attempt to hide a body you are self-conscious about. And try this one on for size. You won't have to 'fish' for complements from anyone about how you look. I can tell you from personal experience that when you are in shape people will be giving you unsolicited complements and praise. I'm 54 years old and I still get complements from younger guys at the gym.

Before I started lifting weights and putting on weight, people made fun of my size, or should I say, my lack of size? I was the guy who got sand kicked in his face. Remember the Charles Atlas ads in the back of old comic books? Well that was me. That all changed when I started gaining muscular body weight. People noticed when I walked by. I was asked if I lifted weights or how much weight could I lift. But I do know somewhat how it feels to go in the opposite direction. I began to gain a little too much of the wrong kind of weight. This resulted in a tummy bulge. I realized that the extra poundage was unnecessary. The weight gain did not come about because I stopped exercising because I never stopped. I just took in too many calories, i.e. I ate too much. I corrected that problem after receiving negative comments.

Here is something else you may not be aware of. You will begin to experience unbelievable amounts of energy. You won't feel a need to grab a banister for support because of sheer exhaustion when walking up or down stairs. So what are the benefits of exercise so far? Well, for one thing you will have a longer life. This life will not only be longer, but it will be a quality life. You'll feel extremely good about yourself. Your self-esteem will skyrocket. Your confidence level will grow. You'll be self-assured, not paranoid and threatened. People will be giving you complements left and right. And it won't stop there. They will be asking you for advice because they want to look just like you! The difference in the way you will feel and in the state of your health will be like the difference between night and day.

The prestigious *New England Journal of Medicine* has stated that diet and exercise can prevent or eliminate type 2 diabetes. According to statistics, 1/3 of American adults or 73 million people either have diabetes or its precursor, impaired fasting glucose. A *National Health and Nutrition Examination Survey* shows that diabetes which was diagnosed rose from 5.1 percent in the years 1988 through 1994 to 6.5 percent from 1999 through 2002.

Starting a weight management program will yield financial benefits in addition to the health and self-esteem benefits. You will no longer have to take out bank loans in order to be able to afford your prescription drugs. The reason is that you will no longer need the medication. Your body will begin to heal itself from the damage caused by excessive weight and by the synthetic drugs you were taking. You also will not be making so many unscheduled visits to the hospital or to the doctor's office.

GETTING STARTED

"Justice delayed is justice denied." Coined by former British Prime Minister William E. Gladstone (1809—1898), this phrase was later quoted and made famous by Martin Luther King, Jr. The principle can be applied to exercise. *Exercise* delayed is *benefits* denied. We can all find excuses for procrastinating. The easiest thing in the world to avoid doing something that needs to be done is to come up with an excuse. And since every excuse we come up with seems reasonable to us, we feel satisfied that we have justified ourselves.

I think the number one excuse that people use to *not* exercise is, "I don't have time." Let's examine this excuse. What is being said in essence is, "I don't have time to engage in physical activity that will strengthen my body and allow it to heal itself. I'd rather continue on my downward spiral, and eventually succumb to mounting medical problems." Are these harsh words? Yes they are. But it is true. You don't have time to exercise but you'll make time to go to the local pharmacist to get your prescription drugs. Why not exercise so that you won't have to be dependent on those drugs which are merely relieving or suppressing symptoms while ignoring the cause of those symptoms? I want to see you as healthy as I am. I want you to *live a God-glorifying life through good health.*

We all have busy schedules. So what do I tell people that bring that excuse to me? Make time! Don't take your health lightly. If we self-destruct our bodies, there's not another one waiting. One body is all we get in this world. If I total my Ford Explorer, I can always replace it. You can't replace your body. You don't have to lift weights like I do. Go walking. Find excuses to walk more. Park your car further from the mall entrance. Climb the stairs instead of always looking for an elevator. Medical experts have determined that walking at a brisk pace could reduce heart disease, stroke, type 2 diabetes, and osteoporosis by 40%! Sure it's going to be tough to begin with. But Rome wasn't built in a day. You've got to remember that your muscles are not used to an exercise routine. They've been under-utilized all these years. Just take it easy when you begin. Your body has to adapt to the new program. Remember, the exercise program will not kill you. Going the way you are by ignoring the problem will.

Years ago a buddy of mine said that he wouldn't go to the gym to work out until he looked a little better. He was worried about how everyone else at the gym would respond to him just because he hadn't lifted weights before. He placed himself in a catch-22 situation. His physique wouldn't improve until he started to weight lift. And he didn't want to weight lift until his physique improved. I guess any excuse is better than none. I told him that those working out in the gym don't busy themselves looking for flaws in each other. They are too busy working to get in shape themselves.

Another excuse is, "I'll start tomorrow or next week." Okay, that may sound reasonable. But it's really not. First of all, tomorrow never comes. It's always today. This is just another form of procrastination. *Never put off until tomorrow what you can do today.* Besides all that, tomorrow isn't promised to you (Read James 4:13–15).

The easiest way to get started exercising is to *just start.* Don't wait for anyone. You are responsible for your own health. Your neighbor, buddy, or your ma and pa aren't. *You are!* There's nothing wrong with wanting to start with someone. But then you are handicapped. *Their excuse becomes your excuse.* After I had the motivation to begin lifting weights, I worked out by myself. I joined a gym, went there religiously, and began getting results. From time to time I did have workout partners. But I never became dependent on them. If my workout buddy didn't or couldn't show up, I was there working out by myself. You have a goal to reach. You have to become self-motivated in order to reach that goal. If you have a walking partner or a lifting partner or a running partner, or whatever, that's good. But if not, so be it. Don't let anything stop you from getting all that God has for you. You *will*, you *can*, and you *must*. I know many people choose walking as their exercise program. That's great. Walking is a weight bearing exercise. Not only is it good for your cardiovascular system, it is also good for bone strength and density. But with walking you will need a backup plan. If you live in the northern areas of the country, the cold and snow may keep you indoors during the winter months. And it may not be feasible to go to the local mall to walk. If you have stairs in your house, walk up and down them several times. There is a personal trainer at Diamond Gym who includes running up and down the stairs as part of his clients' fitness program. But you don't have to run, just walk. And look, it's free. There's no expensive equipment to buy.

If you live in an apartment or house and have no stairs to climb, invest in a stationary bicycle. Although riding a bike doesn't involve weight bearing benefits, it is still great for the cardiovascular system. I would also suggest that you buy two inexpensive dumbbells.

You guys and gals should also take out a subscription to a quality men's and women's fitness magazine respectively. For the women I suggest *Fitness* magazine. I subscribe to this magazine for my wife. It has great articles on the fitness lifestyle. It also lays out diet and nutrition programs and exercise routines. *Fitness* gives women the nuts and bolts of cardio, toning, and strength training programs. There's something there for every woman, no matter what her fitness goals. P.S. I read it myself. Men can try Weider's *Muscle & Fitness* magazine.

OKAY I STARTED, HOW DO I STAY MOTIVATED?

Okay, you got over the first big hurdle. You started your exercise program. You feel excited and giddy. You get an adrenaline rush because you're starting something new—something you've never done before. First of all, never fall into a rut. Don't let your exercise routine become just a routine as days become weeks and weeks turn into months. Keep your mind focused on your objective. And keep the excitement and anticipation there. You're not exercising just to be exercising. And you're not exercising because

I shamed you into it. You are commanded to take care of God's property.

Exercising to get and keep a fit body is a lifetime commitment. If you do it for a while and then stop, your body will return to the sedentary, weak, and overweight state it was in before you started. You are in it for the long haul.

Set short-term goals. "I want to be able to walk one mile nonstop." Keep a journal. Write down your distance and how you feel when you've completed that distance. When I started lifting weights, I kept a workout journey. I wrote down my starting body weight, the exercises I did and their sets and reps (repetitions), and how much weight I used. I wrote down what I ate during the day and how much I weighed when I finished lifting. And then every so often I had photos taken so that I could see my progress. You may also consider taking some measurements. Use a tape measure to get your beginning waist, hip, bust, and upper arm sizes. Write them down. I guarantee that after a short time you will see the progress you're making.

The progress that you make will be self-motivating. You will be pumped up when you see the pounds melting off and your waist and bust shrinking. Your clothes will begin to feel looser. That's what is going to keep you on the program. You're making progress. Your body is changing. You will start to feel better. Deep inside you will know that changes you can't see are happening, too. Your body is beginning to heal itself internally. Rather than feeling so tired and pooped out all the time, you will feel energized. Your sleep pattern will improve, too.

The progress I made lifting weights was mind-blowing. Before I started lifting weights, I was self-conscious because I was really skinny. My height just emphasized that fact. I have a photo of myself in my very first journal. It was taken in October of 1980. I was 22 pounds heavier than when I started. That's motivation right there.

After a while exercise will be an important part of your life. It will become second nature. If I start missing days at the gym for no good reason, my conscience will bother me. If I choose to skip a day, I will make it up some other day that week.

HOW I STARTED LIFTING WEIGHTS

I began lifting weights on a consistent basis in 1978. I was living in an apartment in East Orange, NJ, back then. Prior to 1978 I touched a weight or two at school, but it was only on a couple of occasions. I actually started weight lifting in my living room. I had purchased a 110 pound weight set at Two Guys From Harrison store in Union, NJ (this franchise has since gone out of business). The plates in the weight set that I bought had the vinyl outside coating with the concrete inside. My body weight when I started in 1978 was barely 150 pounds.

When I purchased the weight set, I didn't have anyone to help me carry it. Nevertheless I somehow managed to get the set from the store to my car. Actually I wheeled it to my car in a shopping cart. Before I started to lift weights on a regular basis, I was really weak. I remember years before when my father was living I was helping him do something. I have since forgotten what it was. Apparently I wasn't much help because he accused me of being as "weak as running water." Those were his exact words. Needless to say that hurt my feelings. Dry your eyes, I'm over it now.

When I got to East Orange I remember parking on the opposite side of the street on which I lived. And I think I was about 1/4 block away from my apartment building. I must have presented a pathetic sight struggling to lift/drag that 110 pound set to my building. Thank God it had a working elevator because I lived on the seventh floor.

As time went on I bought more free weights (metal) and a multi-purpose bench. I eventually accumulated several hundred pounds of plates. I exercised regularly in my living room turned gym. I didn't have anyone to work out with so I lifted by myself.

After a while I began to outgrow the weights (I grew stronger). It was at that point that I joined a gym named Guys and Dolls located in Linden, NJ. I was slowly building muscular body weight. Every so often I would have my brother or someone else take physique pictures. When I joined Guys and Dolls gym I began keeping training logs. I still have those journals—all four of them. My very first entry in the very first journal is dated October 28, 1980. I weighed 173 pounds then. By December, 1982 I weighed 191 pounds. By June, 1984 I was up to 204 pounds. In later years I reached a top weight of 212 pounds. Unlike fat, it takes time to build muscle.

In 1982 I joined Diamond Gym located in Maplewood, NJ. The owner/manager is a former IFBB (International Federation of Bodybuilding) competitor John Kemper. Guys and Dolls was too restrictive because it had separate days for men and women. Diamond Gym is co-ed. I was also kind of ashamed of the name of the gym. Silly me. In addition, Diamond Gym had longer hours. It was here that I decided to compete in the Mr. New Jersey bodybuilding show in April, 1982. I dieted down to about 172 pounds. Although I didn't win my weight class, it was a great experience. Almost 20 years later in 2001 I again entered the Mr. New Jersey physique show. Since I was almost 50 years old, I entered the 35 and over class.

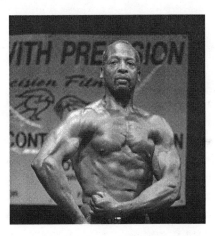

*Author at the 2001 over 35 Mr. New Jersey Bodybuilding show
(Muscle & Fitness; August 2002.)*

From 1978 to the present time I have never looked back. I have consistently trained with weights. When I first started working out in a gym, I trained in the evening after I left work. Several years ago I decided to switch to working out in the morning.

Before my job was eliminated through corporate downsizing, I would go to bed at 8 p.m. and get up at 4 a.m. I typically arrived at the gym at 5:30 a.m. I would work out for an hour. I was on the job by 7:30 a.m. I am currently working from home but I still work out early in the morning. I just don't get up as early.

Before I began lifting weights in 1978, I jogged. My objective was to be able to run a marathon. But when I reached the ten mile mark, I didn't attempt to run any further. I would jog just about every day in Warinanco Park. The distance of the street which went around the park was about two miles. I would run that five times for a total distance of 10 miles. In actuality I can honestly say that I have been exercising consistently for about 30 years.

DISCIPLINE

It has been my experience in both exercising and nutrition that consistency will lead to a disciplined lifestyle. Your life becomes so structured and focused that nothing is able to deter you from your goal. Jack LaLanne, who is still fit and healthy at age 91, said the following, "There are no shortcuts. The truth is you've got to make smart food choices and exercise, not once in a while, but every day." I've done that over the years. That is the reason I am so fit and healthy. Another reason is that I never took any type of medication. No matter what anyone says, there is no better way than God's way. A small investment will yield multiplied results.

Discipline requires that the mind be in total control of the body. This means that despite how you feel (as in I don't feel like walking today) or what the body says (except for injury of course), the mind has total control over the body when it comes to working out. I've gotten up early in the morning when it was cold and snowing outside. I've also gotten up when it was as dark as a closed room with no windows. If you are disciplined enough to eat every day, and several times a day at that, then you can develop the discipline to exercise. Like anything else, anything worth having, or doing, doesn't come easy. But it can still be fun. Effort and fun don't have to be mutually exclusive. Even though working out can put the body through some strain, the benefits will more than compensate for it. That mental fortitude and discipline will keep you on target.

The human body will adapt to a set exercise pattern in time. When that happens, you will stagnate because you will not derive any more benefit from the exercise. The body needs to be challenged. As the body adapts, give it another challenge so that you will continue to make progress. Walk faster, walk further, walk up hills. Carry extra weight in the form of light dumbbells. If you are weight training, vary the sets and reps, and increase the poundage. If you keep the body guessing you will continue to reach higher levels of fitness.

Let me share an inspiring testimonial about the power of discipline. John Wenzel was a top ranked amateur bodybuilder in the 80s and 90s. He had won the overall national bodybuilding championship in 1986. John developed a disciplined lifestyle having started lifting weights after he graduated from college. He began bodybuilding at the Orange, New Jersey YMCA and later trained at John Kemper's Diamond Gym.

In April, 2006 John Wenzel had triple-bypass heart surgery. He is 55 years old. You would think that an operation of this nature coupled with his age would forever end any idea of resuming weightlifting. Not for John. He has a passion for exercise that came about from his disciplined life. John is back at Diamond Gym slowly getting his body back into shape. According to his doctor, he should be able to resume his normal training schedule in about a month and a half. Pointing to his head, John told me that this type of discipline begins here.

No doubt John's fitness level contributed to his speedy recovery. This is a side benefit of exercise. A body which is fit is efficient and better able to deal with any abnormal stress which is placed upon it.

I saw an amazing video on the web recently. It had been broadcast on CNN (Cable Network News) and possibly other television news networks. It showed Pat Robertson who is 74 years old leg pressing 1,000 pounds. The machine he used was an inclined leg press machine. I use this same machine at Diamond Gym. Robertson's physician was a strength trainer. 1,000 pounds total weight equals 500 pounds on each side. This equates to 11–45 pound plates on each side. Take my word for it, that is a lot of weight. The video link is listed at the end of this book

I'm not saying that you have to leg press 1,000 pounds to get in shape but many high profile celebrities including Christians are beginning to realize the value and necessity of exercise.

EXERCISE PROFITETH A LITTLE

> "But refuse profane and old wives' fables, and exercise thyself rather unto godliness. For bodily exercise profiteth little: but godliness is profitable unto all things, having promise of the life that now is, and of that which is to come" (I Timothy 4:7–8).

The use of context in understanding Scripture cannot be emphasized enough. Many well meaning but so *heavenly minded that they are no earthly good* Christians will look at I Timothy 4:8 and tell you that exercising is wrong. I know. I used to be *so heavenly minded that I was no earthly good* (not with exercise, but with other things). But I have since matured as a Christian. Paul, however, is not teaching that exercise is to be avoided. The physical and the spiritual are not mutually exclusive. They must both exist. I have shown that in previous chapters. As long as there is a scriptural balance between the two, God will be well pleased, and you will reap the rewards of an abundant life. When anything is taken to the extreme to the utter exclusion of anything else, problems are unavoidable.

First of all it must be realized that everyone who was contemporary with Paul, both Jew and gentile, did not have any of the modern technological advances that we of the 20th and 21st century take for granted (Review Chapter 2). Therefore the people of Old and New Testament times did not need to have a special exercise period. Their everyday lives involved *strenuous* physical activity. People walked all the time. And many times they were carrying things while they walked. Women undoubtedly carried water containers and their wash back and forth. No one could go to the kitchen faucet to get a glass of water. Neither could they go to the local supermarket to buy bottled water. They had to go a well, bring the water up from the well, and carry it back home. Folks, water is heavy. Try carrying a gallon of bottled water just from the store to the car. That will give you a basic indication of the weight men and women lifted on a daily basis. Weightlifting, jogging, or any of the other types of physical activity common today were unnecessary back then. No doubt a typical day for anyone of the men and women of those ancient times would put most people of today in the hospital. And I am not only talking about our senior citizens. I am referring to our young people also!

I have discovered a wonderful web site for women in general and Christian women in particular. The author of this site is herself a Christian woman who believes as I do concerning nutrition and exercise. I highly recommend this site to all women.[72]

Early Christians and non-Christians also had the benefit of good nutrition. There were no food processing companies to manufacture nutrient deficient products in those days. Neither were there any pharmaceutical companies with highly toxic compounds. Everything grown was organic. Pesticides, herbicides, and insecticides did not exist. Everything that we have in our technically advanced society such as processed, junk foods saturated with sugars and fats, fish containing mercury and other pollutants, veggies grown with the aid of harmful chemicals, and meats containing hormones and antibiotics, were nonexistent back in Bible days.

Okay, let's turn our attention back to I Timothy 4:7–8. Let's take a quick look at I Timothy 4:6 for even more context. "If thou put the brethren in remembrance of these things, thou shalt be a good minister of Jesus Christ, nourished up in the words of faith and of good doctrine, where unto thou hast attained." This epistle or letter was written by Paul to Timothy. "These things" refer to the contents of verses 1 through 5. In verse 7 Paul warns Timothy to avoid "old wives" fables. They are not of God, but of the devil. Timothy is to practice (exercise) godliness. In verse 8 Paul compares the relative merits of physical (bodily) exercise versus practicing godliness. Compared to godliness which benefits Christians in this life, and later in eternity, physical exercise *is* profitable only in this life. Paul *is not* saying that physical exercise does not profit a person at all. Actually the sense of the Greek word translated "little" is, *for a little while.*

Let us also keep in mind that Paul writes that *bodily exercise* 'profits.' It does have its benefits. There can be no valid interpretation or understanding which denies that exercise is beneficial. Back in Bible days, exercise did not have to be emphasized as it does today. Every person in those days, men, women, children, and even the elderly, were physically fit and healthy. There was no health crisis due to toxic chemicals and air pollution and pharmaceutical drugs as there is today. Because of our modern culture, exercise is not a luxury but rather a necessity.

Physical exercise, or anything else for that matter, should not be all consuming. In order of importance it is *godliness* first and exercise second. Don't neglect exercise, but realize its relative value in the total Christian lifestyle. Physical exercise *has* value or merit. It's just that godliness has more. So go ahead and eat right and whip that body into shape. Don't let others run a guilt trip on you. They don't have the Bible on their side but you do. Your Christian ministry or witness cannot go forth if you are always down and out with health problems.

Years ago a seasoned pastor remarked that there is nothing wrong with exercise. He was wearing workout clothing. How many pastors do you know that wear workout clothing and actually work out? Remember what I have drilled over and over again. Today's society is not conducive to good health. It is instead geared to troubling health issues and a shortened, non-quality life. There are subliminal and overt messages all around spreading the gospel of chemically engineered food and living a leisurely and sedentary life. Don't buy into it. You are charged by your Maker to take care of your body.

WHO SHOULD EXERCISE?

In a word, everyone should exercise. Exercise is for every human being on earth. No one is exempt. You are never too young to begin some form of exercise. Children begin exercising as soon as they are able to grasp something and toss it, and again when they begin to crawl and walk. And on the other end of the scale, you are never too old. I've known people who began weight training while in their sixties. I just became acquainted with another senior at Diamond Gym who still lifts weights at the mellow age of 84. I would just caution anyone at any age to check with their physician before they start any type of intense exercise program. And if you are a beginner, take it easy and don't overdo it. You must allow the body time to adapt to exercise after having led a sedentary existence all those years.

Even if an exercise program is begun late in life, the benefits will soon make up for the years of neglect. ". . . Firm, toned muscles, a stronger heart and lungs, increased immunity, and a better quality of life is just a few of the many benefits to be gained by working out regularly. In a study of older adults, researchers found that those who worked out regularly enjoyed long-term improvements in quality of life, self-efficacy, and mood. . ."[73]

Have you heard the adage, "use it or lose it?" It's true. Any part of the body will grow weak from disuse. If you don't use your muscles, not only will you be weak, but as you grow older, they will atrophy. The muscle will be displaced by fat. Fat is metabolically inactive. Muscle on the other hand is metabolically active. It burns calories while at rest. This natural process helps keep the body lean and trim. Inactive muscles are counterproductive to weight loss and weight maintenance.

A person's body weight by itself is not the problem. The problem is that for the majority of people who are overweight or obese, the excess weight is useless fat. When I weighed over 200 pounds, I was overweight according to the standard weight and height charts. That's because those charts don't take into account the amount of muscle a person carries. In reality my body weight, though considerable in comparison to my thin bone structure, was mostly muscle, not fat. Weight lifters, athletes, and bodybuilders carry more lean body mass (muscle) than a sedentary person. Fat is conducive to health problems while muscle equates to fitness.

After I moved into my townhouse in 2003, I decided to take out a life insurance policy that would pay the balance of my mortgage if I were to die. Like anyone else, I wanted the lowest premium possible. I had to submit to a physical examination in order to qualify. My weight then was 204 pounds. When the results of my blood work came back, I qualified for the lowest premium offered. Exercise did that for me.

As a person grows older, muscle will naturally waste away unless some type of exercise is performed. This is why it is imperative that exercise accompany weight management. Proper nutrition will allow the body to burn fat while retaining lean body mass. If weight management is done incorrectly you may lose weight but it will be mostly water and muscle.

Although not as widespread as obesity, underweight individuals are at a significant health risk also. And even though these individuals may appear thin, they can still carry too much body fat. This is especially true for older people. As an individual ages, and leads a largely sedentary life, muscle atrophies. Beginning somewhere around the age of 45, an adult loses approximately 1% of his lean body mass per year. That means that at age 65, that person will have lost 20% of his lean body mass! As an underweight person gets older, he loses muscle mass and gains body fat. If this individual was to have his fat to lean body mass measured, he would find that his body fat percentage is too high for his height and age. Strength training exercise can stop that loss, and even reverse it.

CARDIOVASCULAR EXERCISE

Cardiovascular exercise targets the heart and the blood vessels. "Cardio" comes from the Greek word for heart, "kardia"; "vascular" refers to the blood vessels. Cardiovascular exercise builds heart endurance and increases its efficiency. Walking, jogging, running, dance, and the use of various machines such as the Stairmaster, are all forms of cardiovascular exercise. In addition to increasing the fitness of the cardiovascular system, cardiovascular exercise will reduce body fat levels and help to maintain a lean physique. This type of weight reduction program must be used in conjunction with good nutrition. If not, all you will accomplish is to burn the calories off while exercising and putting them right back on at the dinner table.

Weight reduction means that some foods will have to become history. All bleached foods (white rice, bread, sugar, salt, etc). should be eliminated. They should be replaced with naturally high in fiber whole grains. More fruit and vegetables should be added to the menu. Meats can be organic chicken and turkey breasts, and fish. Dark meat is high in fat so avoid it. I used to love dark meat such as the leg and short joint. I had to give them up though. Drink plenty of water. At least eight, 8 ounce glasses of water should be consumed. More if you are really heavy. And I am not talking about water in your diet sodas either (this will have to be one of the things that will have to become history). The minimum 64 ounces of water per day should be pure water.

Portion control is another important aspect of weight reduction. This is where Americans run into problems. Our typical plate size is 11 to 13 inches. The average plate size in France is 9 inches. The average American eats too much. The plate should not be running over with food. This is not an eating contest. No one is going to be impressed by how much food is gulped down. A portion is much smaller than the typical American eats. For instance, a portion of a lean piece of steak is about the size of a deck of cards.

Contrary to the American standard of three square meals a day, you should eat 5 to 6 *small* meals a day. And *never*, I repeat *never*, skip breakfast. When you skip breakfast or eat just three meals a day, your body perceives it as starvation. The body then slows down its metabolism to conserve fat stores. Eating more frequently lets your body know that you are not starving it, and metabolism increases. Food digestion requires the burning of calories. I've heard people tell me that by eating two or three meals a day they are losing weight. Of that I have no doubt. But if that person was to have his body fat measured, he would find that he is losing muscle, not fat.

Protein requires more stomach acid to break down than either fat or carbohydrate. As a person gets older, the amount of digestive acids that the stomach secretes decreases. Therefore meats should be eaten before fats or carbohydrates. Also a minimum amount of fluid should be drunk with a meal. Water or other liquids tend to dilute stomach acids which lead to incomplete digestion.

Effective cardiovascular exercise requires a frequency of at least three days a week. The American College of Sports Medicine recommends three to five days a week. Start your exercise program off slowly. Remember the race is not given to the swift. You are a novice and your body must become accustomed to cardiovascular training. Start off at a nice, easy pace. In order to derive any benefits from cardiovascular exercise, you should work up to 20 to 60 minutes. Always strive to increase the time. When you have built up endurance (time spent) you can then increase the intensity. How do you do that? By walking or running faster, or by going up hill.

WEIGHT TRAINING

This is a formalized exercise program where specific muscles and muscle groups are targeted with the purpose of strengthening them and preventing atrophy. Weight training exercise is one way towards combating osteoporosis. Although osteoporosis can attack men and women, women are more susceptible. This is especially true of women who are postmenopausal and thin. Men who are thin and underweight don't have enough weight for their bones to support. This can lead to weak and brittle bones. What's the answer? A total body weight lifting program.

A study performed on older women to determine the effect of strength training on bone density yielded surprising results. The women who performed high intensity weight training two days a week were able to increase their bone density by 1%. The control group which consisted of women who did not weight train saw bone density decrease from 1.8% to 2.5%. And look, these results were obtained after only training two days a week. Colossal results from such a small investment in time. This investment could keep you independent of health care aides or family members as long as you live. And it doesn't matter if you live into your 90s, 100s, or beyond.

Combating osteoporosis takes more than just increasing calcium in the diet. One problem with just that approach is that other nutrients must be present in order for the calcium to be absorbed. The consequences of low bone density are evident. Fractures can occur easily and they take a long time to heal. The elderly are especially at risk. The easiest way to stay out of nursing homes and from requiring full time care is to start taking care of yourself *now*. If you don't, and I am not trying to scare you, it's a strong possibility that you'll place a burden on your family later by requiring *their* full-time care. God did not place us on earth to just exist—to just go through the motions. We are here to live and carry out His specific will for our individual lives. His purpose in our lives cannot be fulfilled when we start to decline and wither away in the prime of our lives. ". . . Without resistance exercises to strengthen muscles and bones, most people face a midlife slide into flabbiness and its associated ills. And as we age, strength training becomes even more important to offset age-related declines in muscle and bone mass that can lead to frailty and fracture—the primary reason older adults wind up in nursing homes. . ."[74]

Do I have to join a gym in order to train with weights? No you don't. I began at home. I had bought Arnold Schwarzenegger's book *The Education of a Bodybuilder* to help me learn the different exercises and techniques. If you're not familiar with the different exercises, and you don't have a knowledgeable friend to help you, it might be a good idea to join a gym and get a certified trainer. Or if you can't afford both the gym and the trainer, join a gym and ask other members. It has been my experience that they will be more than happy to assist you. I myself have been asked for assistance down through the years.

As I cautioned with cardiovascular exercise, don't become

overzealous in the beginning. There is plenty of room for injury here. Don't try to use a lot of weight at first either. Slowly build up your strength levels. You can impress your wife or girlfriend when you've become accustomed to the program. And it will also save you a lot of embarrassment too. Take it from someone who knows. It is so easy to let the ego get in the way. Sometimes I try to duplicate my weight lifting accomplishments of some 20 years ago. That can lead to frustration. File the following phrase into your memory banks, *train intelligently*.

Many women are scared off with any mention of weight training. They think that it will turn them into huge, hulking Mr. Olympia contestants. That simply will not happen. God made men and women different. Men were created to carry more muscle than women. Other than increasing bone density, women who train with weights will acquire stronger, firmer, and shapelier muscles. They will begin to lose the flab, especially in problem areas such as the triceps (upper arms). Another concern is that they'll lose their bust. In actuality what will happen is that their pectoral (chest) muscles will be strengthened and become more firm. The weight loss diet will get rid some of the fat, but not much. You will not become flat chested.

Warning to the husbands. A problem may arise if your wife embarks on a weight training program and you don't. She will undoubtedly become stronger as a result. And if there's ever a show of strength guys, you may be embarrassed. You'd better make sure to stay on her good side. Only joking. In reality, a cardiovascular and/or weight lifting program is something that husband and wife can do together.

Weight training has the added benefit of adding muscle. Muscle is metabolically active in that it burns calories. Fat on the other hand does not burn calories. The more muscle that's present translates into more calories burned. And this fat burning activity continues for several hours after weight training. Those of you who are on a weight loss program will benefit tremendously from incorporating weight lifting into your daily routine. What will typically happen is that you will lose a certain amount of fat and gain the same amount of weight in muscle. Although your scale will not show a weight loss, you have succeeded because you have lost fat weight.

I highly recommend adding weight training into your weekly fitness routine even if you do cardiovascular training. And the beauty of weight training is that you don't have to use monstrous pounds of weight in order to reap the benefits. And you needn't be under 40 year old either. Weight training into your 80s and 90s will stop the natural loss of muscle tissue and associated strength levels.

DOCTORS REALIZE IMPORTANCE OF EXERCISE

More and more doctors and professional medical associations are beginning to realize the necessity of exercise. They see America's ever increasing obesity epidemic on a daily basis through personal contact with their patients. The American Academy of Pediatrics wants children's doctors to help be responsible for lifestyle changes in their young patients. The academy also wants the doctors to take an active role in tracking children's physical activity levels in an effort to conquer obesity.

The American Academy of Pediatrics realizes that the key to fighting America's expanding waistline epidemic is by instituting or increasing a child's physical activity level from infancy through the teens. The academy also realizes that parents need to be good role models by setting an example for their children. *Do what I say do not what you see me do* is not a viable option in this crisis.

One of the academy's new policy mandates says that during office visits pediatricians should ask patients and their parents how active they are. Pediatricians should also make sure the children's parents adhere to the academy's guidelines which states that no child under the age of two should watch television. Older children should spend no more than two total hours watching television, playing video games, computer web surfing, etc. The academy is also calling for schools from kindergarten through high school to put mandatory physical education back into their curriculums. As I have written in an earlier chapter neither childhood obesity or mandatory physical education was ever an issue when I was growing up in the 50s and 60s. There *was no* childhood obesity crisis back then but there *was* mandatory physical education in the schools.

Parents have to share in the blame for the rising childhood obesity rates. For one thing, many parents themselves are either overweight or obese. Like parent, like child. Children tend to mimic their parents' behavior and lifestyle. They will copy their parents' food choices and eating habits. Parents are also to blame by giving their children their own personal televisions and video games. And these are in addition to children having their own telephones and cell phones. These electronic devices are addictive. Instead of playing outside they will waste hour after hour with these sedentary and overweight encouraging gadgets.

We all have seen pictures of children and adults who are literally starving to death. We may have seen old file footage of the survivors of the Nazi death camps. Or we may have seen current news broadcasts of starvation in third world countries. The survivors look like living, walking skeletons. We shake our heads in disbelief and horror. But at the same time we think that overweight and obese individuals are normal. We don't look at them as occupying the opposite extreme. But they do. The only difference is that if conditions remain the same, the living skeletons will probably die first. The overweight and the obese are dying a slower death. Medical science has shown that these individuals have a shorter life span than a person of normal weight.

Growing up there was only one television and one radio and one telephone in our house. Personal computers, video games, and cell phones hadn't been invented then. I guess nowadays the kids will report a parent to DYFS if they are not given their own personal television, cell phone, telephone, and computer. I admit that I watched a lot of TV growing up but that was mainly in the evenings after school and after playing outside, and of course, after doing my homework. We weren't allowed to play outside on Sundays so we watched TV then too after church. But back then the TV wasn't in addition to video games, computers, and cell phones.

In Jersey City, we played several games with a small rubber ball. There was punch ball and step ball. Both are variations of baseball. The sidewalk on our street was made up of concrete divided into four squares. Four of us would stand in each square and by using our palms hit the rubber ball to each other. If I remember correctly, the objective was to get the other person to miss the ball or to hit it outside the squares or on the line. We also played giant steps and tag. The boys would also play a game called tops. This game was played in the street with bottle tops within a series of chalk drawn lines. We also rode our scooters. We propelled ourselves with one leg. We also roller skated in the street and on the sidewalk and rode bicycles.

As you can see, we were pretty active. Although we had our share of sodas and pastries, those extra calories were burned off in no time. You could count on one hand the kids who were considered to be fat back then. They were rare.

EXERCISE AND CANCER

It is well known that a change in lifestyle is a must to prevent or drastically reduce the risk of cancer. The first thing that should be done is to stop smoking. The next thing is to eliminate or reduce as much as possible second hand smoke. After those changes have been made, the next step is to put in place healthier eating habits. All white products should be removed from the menu (sugar, bread, salt, rice). Next step is to replace all fast and processed and refined foods with whole (natural) foods. What is not as well known is that exercise also reduces the risk of cancer.

A recent write-up in the *British Medical Journal* explored the relationship between exercise and cancer risk. It was noted that several factors had a direct bearing on the risk of cancer. These factors are:

1. Cardiovascular capacity
2. Pulmonary capacity
3. Bowel movement

4. Hormone levels
5. Energy balance
6. Immune system function
7. Antioxidant defense and
8. DNA repair. Daily exercise improved these factors which lessens the risk of cancer.

People who exercise have half the risk of developing bowel cancer than those who lead a sedentary life. Using laboratory mice on running wheels, it was discovered that fewer and smaller skin tumors developed. It is also interesting to note that reducing body fat levels produced a reduction in the number of tumors.

A strength training study was done with 54 women ages 30 through 50 to determine its effect on several risk factors which can lead to breast and colon cancer. The study lasted 9 months and measured changes in body fat percentage, waist size, fasting insulin, fasting glucose, and insulin-like growth factor I (IGF-I). There was no nutritional diet associated with this study. The women used weights to strength train only twice a week.

This strength training regimen produced an increase in lean body mass (muscle), and reductions in body fat percentage and fasting insulin and glucose levels. Amazingly, it only took 15 weeks to achieve these measurable results. A strength training program can also be implemented to help prevent a recurrence of breast and colon cancer.

One of the primary effects of exercise is that it pushes insulin levels down. This is good. There have been several studies undertaken throughout the world to determine why centenarians live as long as they do. The study subjects varied in lifestyles. Some smoked, others didn't. Some exercised while others didn't. Some also drank, others didn't. The only common denominator between all centenarians studied was that *they all had low insulin levels for their age*. At one time it was thought that the only purpose of insulin was to lower the body's blood sugar levels. It is now known that the primary purpose of insulin is to store excess nutrients. Insulin stores carbohydrates. Some bodybuilders inject themselves with insulin in order to build bigger muscles and to store protein. Insulin also stores magnesium. Centenarian studies have shown that insulin sensitivity is the major indicator for lifespan. If a person's cells are not sensitive, insulin levels skyrocket. Hence we have the term insulin resistance. Insulin resistance is the cause of the disease of aging. The symptoms of this disease of aging are what the medical profession looks upon as the disease itself—cancer, osteoporosis, diabetes, heart disease, obesity, etc.

Whenever the body's cells are exposed to insulin, they become more resistant. This is normal and cannot be stopped. The rate however can be controlled. When insulin resistance increases, we age. Remember from the centenarian study that all participants had low insulin levels. It is believed that we can push the boundaries of life even further than 100 or 110. Centenarians should be able to live to 120, 130, or even 140 years!

Here is the problem with today's overweight and obese population. America is overdosing on sugar. Addiction to regular and diet sodas, cakes, cookies, and other pastries, as well as artificial sweeteners which in one form or another is in just about all processed food is at an all time high. When sugar is ingested, it immediately raises the body's blood sugar level. Insulin skyrockets and the cells become more insulin resistant. This process continues to put the body at risk for the symptoms of aging such as cancer and osteoporosis. This is turn reduces the lifespan.

As far as insulin is concerned, carbohydrates are either fibrous or they are not fibrous. The fruit sugar fructose is not fibrous. When a person drinks Tropicana orange juice his blood sugar skyrockets. When a person eats an orange he is still ingesting the fructose but the fiber from the pulp prevents an insulin surge (stops the blood sugar from skyrocketing). An orange is much better for you than orange juice. The body sees a white potato as a large glob of sugar. It contains no fiber so your blood sugar jumps just as if you had eaten a large lump of sugar. I am not advocating avoidance of fruit juice and white potatoes. But I would recommend that the fruit be eaten much more often. You should definitely avoid drinking all fruit *drinks*. I would also recommend that sweet potatoes be eaten in place of white potatoes. They are much more nutritious for you. Fructose (fruit sugar) and lactose (milk sugar) will raise blood sugar levels just as quickly as sucrose (table sugar).

Whenever insulin rises (or blood sugar levels become elevated), fat is not being burned. When the body doesn't burn fat, it stores it. This is what happens to the overweight and obese. Their insulin levels are constantly being elevated and they store more and more fat.

Experiments have shown conclusively that resistance (weight) training will increase insulin sensitivity much more effectively than aerobic (running, jogging) training. Insulin sensitivity is determined by how blood gets to an area of the body. The greater the blood flow to a muscle, the greater the sensitivity. Whenever I lift weights, I make it a point to make sure that blood is circulating in the muscle that I am about to train. I do this by doing the exercise with a very light weight. Once the target muscle is warm, i.e. a lot of blood is circulating, I can use heavier weights.

As with good nutrition, there are no negatives in regard to exercise. You can't go wrong, and unlike the stock market, there are no losses, only gains. I would recommend putting in place a good weight training program along with the cardiovascular training (walking, running, or jogging). As you can see a little produces a lot when it comes to overall results and fitness level.

EXERCISE AND THE FLU

There just seems to be no end to the benefits of regular exercise. University of Illinois researchers conducted a study to discover the role of exercise in mice that had contracted influenza (the flu). After they had the flu, the mice were exercised 20 to 30 minutes a day for four days. The exercise program was stopped after flu symptoms appeared in the mice. The result of this study was that the mice that were exercised did not die from the flu. What would the results have been if the mice were exercised regularly prior to the flu exposure?

It is well known that exercise increases blood circulation. This allows the body's immune elements to circulate more quickly and efficiently on a search and destroy mission. Any illness is halted dead in its track before it can spread causing harm throughout the body. This is a natural alternative to flu vaccines.

To date, Americans rely on flu vaccinations for protection. Unknown to them is the fact that these vaccines contain mercury and aluminum. Both aluminum and mercury are toxic, and aluminum has been linked to Alzheimer's disease. These toxins slowly build in the body's soft tissues resulting in medical problems down the road. Exercise is the logical alternative. There is no downside to exercise and the results are always positive.

I am not sure, but I may have had a flu shot many years ago. Even if I did, I have had none since. While working for Elizabethtown Gas Company, my coworkers would march every year to get their flu vaccinations. Even though the vaccinations where free, I passed on the opportunity. I have never contracted the flu. And unlike the mice in the study, I have exercised consistently for decades. That was my flu vaccination. Why have aluminum and mercury pumped into your veins every year when you can go the natural route and not poison your body? And unlike the flu shot, you are guaranteed results.

Again, it was only the grace of God which prevented me from getting the free flu vaccinations all that time. Back then I had no idea how dangerous the vaccines were. As a matter of fact, I didn't know they were dangerous at all. It was the same with prescription drugs. And it was the same with aspirin. After awhile I just stopped taking aspirin. I haven't a clue as to why.

Influenza vaccines are not even a band aide for the virus. They are totally useless. The only proven remedy for the flu and other illnesses is an adherence to God's maintenance plan for your body. Eat His whole foods and exercise. It's as simple as that. I've explained it all in the current and preceding chapters. You too can reject man's deadly answer to influenza just as I have, and remain flu free.

Closing Thoughts

This has been a fascinating and rewarding journey. In the course of doing the research I have learned a lot. Much of what I have learned is not something that is widely publicized through the media. The truth about the pharmaceutical, dairy, and food industries is highly secretive. Now I know why. If the American public knew and fully understood the implications of what these powerful industries were really doing to them through their products, they would be up in arms.

It is just because of what I have learned while writing this book that I have made some major health changes in my life. I pray that you too will follow in my footsteps. I have never taken prescription or nonprescription drugs. (I didn't avoid these drugs because I knew that they were bad. I didn't know that until I began doing the research for this book). I was never prescribed these drugs because I never had health issues. I thank God for that.

My education concerning pharmaceutical drugs began quite by accident. I was over my mother's house one day and there was an infomercial on one of the satellite channels. This infomercial captivated my attention. It was Kevin Trudeau advertising his landmark book *Natural Cures "They" Don't Want You To Know About*. Kevin was revealing things about the pharmaceutical companies that I kind of suspected, but didn't know for sure. I knew intuitively that he was right. And I also knew that he had insider knowledge that the general public did not have. I went to my local Barnes & Noble bookstore and purchased the book the very next day. That single book has changed my life and perspective completely. In fact, it has changed my life so thoroughly that I purchased an additional two copies to give away as gifts.

Something else which has really impacted my life is the truth about the food industry. The operation of the meat industry is especially heinous. I know that God made animals subordinate to man. However, the fact that animals are lower doesn't give man the authority to abuse them. Animals are inhumanely treated and tortured in the process of slaughtering. This is exactly what happens to cows, chickens, turkeys, pigs, and other animals which wind up on America's lunch and dinner plates (Read *The Jungle* by Upton Sinclair).

After I found out how animals were treated prior to being slaughtered, I had second thoughts about eating meat. Don't misunderstand my position now. I am no animal rights activist. But what I read disgusted me. When I began writing this book I was a meat eater. But after reading about the hormones, antibiotics, pesticides, and other harmful chemicals animals were subjected to, and how residual amounts remain in the meat we buy, I decided to purchase organic meats only. Shortly afterwards I became a vegetarian.

The sad truth about the dairy industry also came to my attention. I read that cows were injected with growth hormone that causes all kinds of problems both to the cows and to milk drinkers. On November 8, 2005 I bought the book *The Wellness Revolution* by Paul Zane Pilzer. I learned from this book that cows are given bovine growth hormone (BGH). Mr. Pilzer wrote that milk tainted with BGH is the cause of allergies, gas, constipation, obesity, cancer, and other diseases. I noticed that I had experienced serious gas and bloating after drinking milk. It was then that I substituted soy milk for cow's milk. I didn't have any more gas or bloating. Now I drink Silk's soy milk exclusively.

Now that I have become a total vegetarian, and eat no meat or fish or any dairy product whatsoever, I feel great. And what's even more amazing is the fact that I don't miss eating meat. And I have been eating meat for almost 55 years. I decided not to eat fish because our waters are becoming increasingly more polluted. And there is still the mercury to contend with. To be honest, I don't believe for a minute that scientists have a complete knowledge of the scope of this problem.

Despite becoming a vegetarian, I am still able to work out hard in the gym. My energy levels are great and my strength hasn't left me. As a matter of fact, even though I have been a vegetarian for less than a month to date, I can honestly say that overall, I feel better than I did before. There is a side benefit to my becoming a vegetarian. It is financial. Meat was the single most expensive item in my food budget. Now that I no longer eat meat, my weekly food bill is actually lower even though I buy organic.

If you make the choice to become a vegan (no meat, fish, or dairy), you have to make sure that you have a source of vitamin B12. This particular B vitamin is found almost exclusively in meat and dairy products. I drink plenty of Silk soy milk, which is fortified with vitamin B12. It is also in the multivitamin that I take.

I know what you're thinking. You don't think that you could never give up eating meat. If I had a dollar for all the times I said I never would do something, I would be a very rich man. To tell you the truth, if someone had told me at the beginning of this year that I would become a vegetarian in a few months, I would have thought that he was out of his mind. Just goes to show you, *never* say never! Even without meat, I still look forward to eating. And I yet enjoy my meals. But now I rest in the fact that my body is a lot healthier (I am not taking in the hormones and antibiotics from nonorganic animal meat) and I am able to glorify God even more through it.

The only concern I had about giving up meat was getting adequate protein. I always thought that meat was *the* major source of protein and that all other sources merely supplemented it. Boy was I wrong. Being a bodybuilder for almost 30 years, I had grown accustomed to eating at least one meal with meat. I have since learned that the protein in vegetables, brown rice, beans, soy milk, and other natural products is more than sufficient. Since I still eat 5 to 6 small meals a day, I get more than enough protein. I have since changed my mind about the amount of protein I need too. One gram of protein for every 2 pounds of body weight is enough for me. When I carried over 200 pounds of body weight, I ate one gram of protein for every pound of body weight.

Another thing that I have changed is now I buy everything organic. I do my shopping at Whole Foods. All fruits, vegetables, beans, yams, sweet potatoes, etc. are organic. Although slightly more expensive than non organic foods, it is worth the extra expense to me. I look at it this way. When I ask myself how much my health is worth, the answer always is that is priceless.

After I learned what I did about microwave ovens (See Chapter 5), I don't use them anymore. I purchased an electric convection oven which I use to cook yams and sweet potatoes. I cook my brown rice on the stove. And I now eat my vegetables raw. This ensures that I get all the nutrients that are in them. I pour either olive oil or flaxseed oil on them. It's great. Of course I still supplement with vitamins and minerals.

There used to be a saying, "What you don't know won't hurt you." I'm not sure if that was ever true. But I know it definitely isn't true when it pertains to health. The truth about the addictiveness of nicotine, though known and planned for by Big Tobacco, was carefully hidden from the public. The fact that millions of cigarette smokers were ignorant of that fact didn't protect them from lung cancer and other serious health problems. The same is true about Big Pharma and the food and dairy industries. The fact that the FDA knew about the problems with Vioxx but chose to keep silent about them did not prevent the deaths of the thousands of people who were prescribed Vioxx by their doctors.

No industry will ever willingly give up billions of dollars in sales just because its products contribute to or cause serious harm to consumers. In the words of Kevin Trudeau, 'it's all about the money.' In the words of God, "For the love of money is the root of all evil. . . " (I Timothy 6:10a). The dairy industry will continue to sponsor high profile athletes and celebrities with their fake "milk" moustaches to tout the health benefits of milk. This is in spite of the fact that dairy cows are injected with dangerous growth hormone to make it possible for them to give more milk than God ever intended them to. And let's not forget that these cows are fed everything but what God created them to eat—grass. Cows are also given antibiotics to combat infections.

The animals intended for slaughter are not even protected by the Animal Welfare Act. Animals such as dogs, cats, and birds are protected by law from being treated inhumanely, but cows, pigs, and chickens are not. Besides being tightly packed in overcrowded pens, cattle are fed everything and anything to get them fat.

> . . . Here the animals are fed a diet designed for one purpose only-to fatten them up as cheaply as possible. This may include such delicacies as sawdust laced with ammonia and feathers, shredded newspaper (complete with all colors of toxic ink from the Sunday comics and advertising circulars), "plastic hay," processed sewage, inedible tallow and grease, poultry litter, cement dust, and cardboard scraps. . . [75]

You know the old saying, "You are what you eat?" Well you may be eating beef that has been fed trash which by no stretch of the imagination resembles food. And don't forget the insecticides, hormones, and antibiotics they ingest. Their "food" is so bad that the animals have to be deceived into eating it by having artificial flavors and aromas added to it. You can be certain that a consistent diet of this meat will cause medical problems. It's just a matter of time. Do you have an undiagnosed medical problem? It may stem from the beef you are eating.

When Americans drink milk or eat meat, they are also ingesting hormones, antibiotics, insecticides, and Lord knows what other deadly chemicals. And doctors are scratching their heads wondering where all the cancer is coming from? I'm like the blind man in John 9:25. "He answered and said, Whether he be a sinner or no, I know not: one thing I know, that, whereas I was blind, now I see." I was once blind to how the pharmaceutical, food, meat and dairy industries conducted their business. But through research my eyes have been opened. Now I see! These industries will never again have me purchase their poisoned products wrapped in glitter and gold. What about you?

Because of what my research has revealed concerning the pharmaceutical, food, and dairy industries, I don't trust them anymore. They are caught in the powerful grip of profit. "For the love of money is the root of all evil. . . " They will never acknowledge the dangers, or even possible dangers, of their products and/or processes to their customers. As I have said in previous chapters, these companies are in business to make money for their shareholders. It, however, is one thing to make money, and something else entirely when it is done unethically. When chemicals are added to foods to make the consumer fatter and to get them addicted, ethics are thrown out of the window. I also don't trust the Food and Drug Administration (FDA). Since they seem to have a vested interest in the pharmaceutical and food industries, they can't be expected to make impartial judgments when it comes to consumer health.

America is being seduced by food and a sedentary life brought upon us by machines. There is nothing wrong with food and there is nothing wrong with machines. Food does become a problem when it begins to control us, and not the other way around. Eating too much of it can lead to gluttony. This is a sin. "For the drunkard and the glutton shall come to poverty: and drowsiness shall clothe a man with rags" (Proverbs 23:21). America has to get away from processed food. We have to go back to the good old days and spend more time in the kitchen preparing nutritious meals for our families. The only other alternative is health problems and an early grave. Machines and devices have taken complete control over our lives. They remind me of an early Twilight Zone episode where machines "rebelled" against their owner. But instead of rebelling against us, we are allowing machines to make us weak and lazy and overly dependent on them.

Going back to the good 'ole days of better quality food and more physical activity is a no-brainer to me. In order to live a God-glorifying life through good health, serious changes to our current lifestyles have to be made. I made the necessary changes with no reservations and I have no regrets. I am just sorry that I didn't realize it a lot sooner. Oh well, better late than never!

I guess you are wondering if you have to do everything I did in order to be healthy. There is an old proverb which says that all great journeys begin with the first step. Take it one step at a time. This is something that you have to want to do. I got committed from what God's Word said and from what my research has revealed. I wanted to change. My personality type is such that I am able to take giant steps, or in some instances, one great leap. You may be only able to take small steps. That's alright. You do what you are capable of doing. I just encourage you to take the first step, no matter how small.

The first step I would encourage you to take is to gradually remove all white, processed food from the diet. This includes sugar, table salt, bread, rice, etc. Replace the white bread with whole grain bread and replace the white rice with brown rice. I also recommend replacing white potatoes with sweet potatoes (please leave the skin on). Sweet potatoes contain almost four times the RDA (recommended daily allowance) of beta-carotene, are high in fiber, and contain vitamin B6 and the mineral potassium. If possible, go the organic route. The next thing I would do is to gradually stop eating all fast foods. Take the time to eat healthy, home-prepared meals. God didn't make you to feed your body trash. Why do you think it is called "junk food"? Keep in mind that you are a son of God. That signifies that you are a son of a king. The king eats nothing but the best. The so-called "food" manufactured by food companies whose only god is the almighty buck certainly doesn't qualify as "best." "Best" food is food as close to its natural state as possible. That means the way you find it in nature.

You don't have to become a vegetarian like I did, but I would definitely eat only organic meat. I recommend skinless chicken and turkey breasts and fish. Stay away from veggie burgers because they are processed, and sugars and food addictive chemicals are added. Increase the amount of fruit and vegetables that you eat. If you are anything like I was, you are not getting the suggested 5 to 7 recommended servings daily. Try eating your vegetables raw. If you prefer not to, I would recommend steaming them.

It's unfortunate that due to today's nutrient depleted soil, fruits and vegetables don't have the amount of minerals and vitamins that they had when our grand and great grandparents were growing up. It has been estimated that today's produce can have up to 60 percent less vitamins and minerals than it had just 30 years ago. Do you realize how many vegetables you would have to eat in order to get the equivalent amount of nutrients that your grandparents got? Cooking further removes vital nutrients (they wind up in the water).

By gradually eliminating all processed food from the diet, and increasing the intake of fruit and vegetables, you are adding more fiber. This is a good thing. The additional fiber along with the protein helps to fill you up. This encourages you not to overeat (good for weight control). Add nuts to your diet. My favorite nuts are almonds and pecans. But brazil nuts and walnuts are good, too. Get the raw, unsalted kind. Nuts contain the healthy fats.

Whether you become a vegetarian or not, try to eat at least one serving of cruciferous vegetables every day. Broccoli, brussels sprouts, cabbage, cauliflower, and kale are classified as cruciferous. These particular vegetables are great cancer fighters. They contain the phytonutrient isothiocyanates which has the ability to increase the capacity of the liver to detoxify carcinogens (cancer causing agents). These vegetables also protect against vision impairment from cataracts and macular degeneration.

Drink more water. How do you know when you are drinking enough water? Instead of the once popular standard of eight 8 ounce glasses a day, determine need by the color of your urine. If your urine is pale to light yellow, you are adequately hydrated. If your urine is dark yellow, or worse yet, an orange color, you are not drinking nearly enough water. I am talking about pure, uncontaminated and unmixed water. Give up drinking all sodas, including diet sodas. Adequate water intake aids in body fat removal which means healthy weight control.

The best way to lose or maintain body weight is by eating smaller meals frequently throughout the day. The American standard of three squares a day is not the best way to eat. Eating this infrequently with so much time between meals encourages the body's metabolism to slow down which in turn makes it harder to lose weight. This means that your body burns calories at a slower rate. The body perceives that it is starving. By merely reducing calories in an attempt to lose weight, precious lean body mass, i.e., muscle, will be sacrificed instead, and body fat retained.

It has been discovered that the body will burn up to 10% more calories when given frequent, smaller meals. It also places less stress on the heart. A large meal causes the heart to beat up to 30 times faster than a smaller meal. This increases the risk of having a heart attack. Also frequent, smaller meals stabilize your blood sugar level. I recommend eating 5 to 6 small meals per day. Each meal should include a protein source such as nuts (almond, walnut, pecan, etc). Eating small, frequent meals is known as grazing. And remember, portion control is also important. Frequent eating is not a license to indulge in huge portion sizes.

By taking it one step at a time, you are slowly replacing poisons with God created healthy whole and natural food. This not only provides the basic materials the body needs to stay healthy, but also allows the body to heal itself from the years of chemical ingestion. And when you institute a consistent exercise program, you will find that you may not need the harmful pharmaceutical medications you are presently taking. By not having to depend on toxic drugs, the body will begin to recover even further.

Once you begin implementing the steps that are required to live a God-glorifying life through good health, you will experience the abundant life in Christ. There is a downside to all this good health though. You will not be able to call in sick for work because you will not get sick. Sorry about that. But other than that, there is no downside. You will feel so good that you may consider running the next Boston marathon or challenging your son to a one-on-one basketball game. Yes, you will experience that level of health and well being. This higher level of health translates into additional years of life. And those additional years will be quality years. I'd say that it's well worth the effort, wouldn't you?

Your entire way of thinking will change. You will not think of yourself as old and weak. Neither will you expect to get arthritis, Alzheimer's disease, osteoporosis, senility, or any of the dozens of other ailments society usually associates with senior citizens. You will expect to live a long, abundant, and productive life. Your future will not be spent in a nursing home or in a wheel chair. Do you know what else? You won't have to worry about budgeting for various medications. Do you know why? Your body will be so healthy, the way God intended it to be, that you won't need any pharmaceutical drug as long as you live. Besides, I know that you have much better things to do with your hard earned money than buying toxic drugs. *God does not desire that His people be enslaved by drugs.*

> "Beloved, I wish above all things that thou mayest prosper and be in health, even as thy soul prospereth" (III John 2).

After all I've said you still don't think that you can do it? Yes you can. It all begins with a healthy mental attitude and outlook. Where the mind leads, the body must follow. And you are not alone. Everything that you do should be done *through* Christ. If this program is tackled through Christ, it can't fail.

> "I can do all things through Christ which strengtheneth me" (Philippians 4:13).

Don't believe the devil's lie concerning your body and your life here on earth. He is a liar because that is his nature. "Ye are of your father the devil, and the lusts of your father ye will do. He was a murderer from the beginning, and abode not in the truth, because there is no truth in him. When he speaketh a lie, he speaketh of his own: for he is a liar, and the father of it" (John 8:44).

HEALTH AND FITNESS: THERE IS A DIFFERENCE

I think that if one were to conduct a survey concerning 'health' and "fitness," the consensus would be that the terms are interchangeable or synonymous. In reality there is a difference between being healthy and being fit. A person can be fit but not healthy. Conversely, a person can be healthy but not fit. A real life example will serve to illustrate the difference between the two. I once knew a bodybuilder who was fit, but not healthy. Although he lifted weights just like I do, he also smoked cigarettes. His extremely fit body could not mitigate the harmful effects of nicotine. There is an abundance of amateur and professional athletes who take performance enhancing drugs. Look at what's happening in baseball. Unfortunately this epidemic is not limited to baseball. These athletes are very fit, but the toxic drugs are compromising their health.

How do we obtain health? How do we get fit? Getting healthy involves a lifestyle choice. The choice has to be made to provide the body with nutrients that God, not Satan, has placed on earth. Whole organic foods are the only foods that can give you a healthy body. A whole food diet will provide the body with all the minerals, vitamins, fats, protein, fiber, and carbohydrates the body needs. These substances will include plenty of antioxidants which are needed to rid the body of health destroying free radicals. Free radicals are dangerous. It is because of free radicals that cancer is able to thrive.

It is simple to tell the difference between the foods that Satan has created and those provided by God. Satan's foods are those that have been changed, stripped of nutrients, or bleached. Foods are changed by having foreign chemicals such as sweeteners, MSG, preservatives, and artificial flavors and colorings added to them. Foods such as wheat, sugar, and rice are stripped of vital nutrients to give them 'eye appeal.' The result of this nutrient stripping is white bread and rolls, white sugar, and white rice. Processed foods such as crackers, cookies, and pastries have enticing colors added to them. Any food that has been processed is Satan's counterfeit. The food that God has given mankind is found in nature.

Examples are organic beef and chicken and organically grown fruit and vegetables.

We have to be both healthy and fit in order to enjoy the abundant life that Christ has promised us. We have to eat nutritious natural foods and exercise our bodies. There is no other way and there is no shortcut. Do one without the other and you will compromise the temple of the Holy Ghost. Willful violation of God's natural laws will invoke the natural law of consequences. No matter how much you pray before you leave the house, you still have to look both ways before crossing the street. If not I guarantee that you will suffer the consequences (possibility of getting struck by a fast moving vehicle and getting to see Jesus prematurely).

RESTAURANTS AND A HEALTHY DIET

How many times have you heard someone say, "I don't eat everyone's cooking?" Maybe you have said it yourself. I'd say that 99.9 percent of the time that statement is inaccurate. When food is eaten in a restaurant, you are eating someone else's cooking. And not only are you eating someone else's cooking, but that someone else is a total stranger to you.

How about it? Can anyone maintain a healthy diet away from home? First of all allow me to clarify what I mean when I talk about restaurants. I am not including your local pizza joint, neither am I including fast food restaurants such as McDonald's, KFC, Popeye's, Burger King, etc. I am though including such franchises as Red Lobster, Captain D's and the Cracker Barrel. Personally I was never a big eating out person. For me eating at home is the rule while going to a restaurant is the exception.

Since I am now fully aware of the toxic chemicals which are used in seemingly harmless food, I am cautious. When I do find myself in a restaurant, I try to make as intelligent a choice as I can. I can do this and still enjoy my food. If I weren't a vegetarian I would stay away from all meats with the exception of fish. The fish would be either baked or broiled. I would refuse all sauces (they are probably loaded with MSG and saturated or trans fat). I would have my vegetables steamed. I would just suggest that you do the best you can.

Avoid all fast food franchises entirely. There is absolutely no reason to patronize these anti-health establishments. Naturally if you happen to be out of town for business or pleasure, you have no choice but to eat out. I suggest making an informed choice as to what's on the menu. I would also question your server as to food preparation. I would let him (or her) know that you are on a restricted diet (a diet restricted to natural food). And don't hesitate to let your server know what you do and do not want. After all, you are a paying customer and they are there to satisfy you.

In the final analysis, you are an individual. Completely abandoning your restricted diet once in a while will not destroy your health. But you control your diet. Don't let it control you. Here's to that occasional cheat meal.

TO WHOM DO I OWE THE PLEASURE?

God desires for you to have a fit and healthy body in order that you might prosper. So it is to Him that you first owe the pleasure of a healthy temple. You next owe the pleasure to yourself. And lastly, you owe the pleasure to those who depend on you. This includes but is not limited to your family, co-workers, community, etc. So, in order of priority it is God, yourself, and others.

No one lives in a vacuum. The state of our lives and health will inevitably affect others. To neglect that aspect is an act of selfishness. For me to purposely neglect my health means that I won't be able to adequately provide for my wife. When my health deteriorates I become susceptible to sickness and disease. This in turn will bring grief to my mother (she worries a lot about her children). This unnecessary grief and worry will add stress to my mother and possibly trigger a heart attack. Do you see my point? I don't want it on my conscience that I failed my family. Knowledge is empowerment. By living in the fullness of God's joy by taking care of His temple, you automatically fulfill your responsibility to others. This is the ultimate experience that a Christian can have. The spirit man is growing and maturing while the physical man has achieved the pinnacle of achievement. In actuality, you don't even have to worry about "self." When you please God and others, you automatically please yourself. So let's revise "To whom do I owe the pleasure?" The answer is to God and then others (family, community, etc).

Must Read / *Watch* / *Visit*

Robbins, John. *Diet For A New America*. H.J. Kramer, 1987.

Trudeau, Kevin. *Natural Cures "They" Don't Want You To Know About*. Alliance Publishing Group, 2004.

Pilzer, Paul Zane. *The Wellness Revolution*. John Wiley & Sons, 2002.

Schlosser, Eric. *Fast Food Nation* Harper's Perennial, 2002.

Super Size Me DVD

Prescription For Disaster DVD

Sweet Misery: A Poisoned World DVD

WEB SITES:

www.mercola.com
www.consumerhealth.org/articles/display.cfm
www.gillistriplett.com/healing/articles/belly.html
www.geocities.com/reflectpool/body.html
www.byregion.net/articles-healers/Hunza_Diet.html
www.godkind.org/health.html
www.cbn.com/communitypublic/shake.aspx
www.bibleevidences.com/medical.htm
http://www.foodrevolution.org/index.htm
http://www.ultrametabolism.com
http://www.vegsource.com
www.themeatrix.com
www.mercola.com/2005/apr/13/cancer_risk.htm
http://www.goveg.com/factoryFarming_cows_flesh.asp

1. (Strong's # 5198)

2. (Strongs's # 2137)

3. (www.thedailycamera.com/livingarts/religion/25pdiet.html)

4. (www.mercola.com/2006/may/18/americans_are_
   sicker_than_most_of_the_world.htm)

5. (www.fluoridealert.org/fluoridation.htm; Dr. J. William
   Hirzy, Senior Vice-President, Headquarters Union, US
   Environmental Protection Agency, March 26, 2001)

6. (www.holistichealthtools.com)

7. (www.holistichealthtools.com/water1.html)

8. (Take A Hint From the Hunzas: Diet Is Key to Health, Vitality;
   www.byregion.net/articles-healers/Hunza_Diet.html)

9. (www.unec.net/of_interest/HunzaDietBread.htm)

10. (http://news.bbc.co.uk/1/low/world/americas/4501646.stm)

11. (www.walking.about.com/od/healthbenefits)

12. (http://www.kidshealth.org)

13. (Stress: Why You Have It and How It Hurts Your Health;
    www.mayoclinic.com/health/stress/SR00001)

14. (http://news.bbc.co.uk/1 /low/world/americas/4501646.stm)

15. (www.aricept.com)

16. (www.newstarget.com/010315.html)

17. (www.newstarget.com/010315.html)

18. (*Alternatives For the Health-Conscious Individual*; April, 2006- Vol. 11, #10)

19. (www.csun.edu/~vceed002/health/docs/tv&health.html)

20. (www.mercola.com/2000/mar/13/television_fast_food.htm)

21. (*The Star-Ledger*; Thursday, April 6, 2006; pg. 3)

22. (*Natural Cures "They" Don't Want You To Know About*, pg. 193)

23. (http://www.kff.org/entmedia/entmedia052406nr.cfm)

24. (Beating the Food Giant; from the chap-
    ter entitled "The Natural Revolution")

25. (*The Next Millionaires*; pgs. 42–43)

26. (*Dirty Secrets of the Food Processing Industry*; www.
    consumerhealth.org/articles/display.cfm)

27. (Dirty Secrets of the Food Processing Industry)

28. (*The Powerfood Nutrition Plan*; pg. 155)

29. (http://news.bbc.co.uk/1/low/world/americas/4501646.stm)

30. (*The Powerfood Nutrition Plan*; pg. 155)

31. (Beating the Food Giants)

32. (www.womentowomen.com/nutritionandweightloss/splenda)

33. (*The Wellness Revolution*; pg. 81)

34. (*Dirty Secrets of the Food Processing Industry*)

35. (The Star-Ledger; Thursday, April 13, 2006)

36. (*The Star-Ledger*; Thursday, April 13, 2006)

37. (*The Powerfood Nutrition Plan*; pgs. 93, 94)

38. (*Alternatives*; Summer, 2006)

39. (www.nutrition4health.org/nohanews/nnsp00_msg.htm)

40. (www.nutrition4health.org/nohanews/NNSp00_msg.htm)

41. (www.consumerhealth.org/articles/display.cfm)

42. (www.consumerhealth.org/articles/display.cfm)

43. (www.fda.gov/fdac/features/2000/300_soy.html)

44. (www.bellaonline.com/articles/art15448.asp)

45. (www.bellaonline.com/articles/art15448.asp)

46. (www.truthaboutsplenda.com/factvsfiction/index.html)

47. (www.hps-online.com/foodprof1.htm)

48. (*Food Labels: How Do You Know Who's Telling The Truth?* Sarah Levi, Community Education Coordinator for Project mana)

49. (www.goveg.com/factoryFarming_cows_flesh.asp)

50. (*Death by Medicine*; Specific Drug Iatrogenesis: Antibiotics)

51. (www.gillistriplett.com/healing/articles/belly.html)

52. (Amy Patel M.S., M.P.H., *Is Your BMI Making You Sick?* AOL Diet & Fitness; June 23, 2006)

53. (3/1/2004, Vol. 159 Issue 5; pgs. 454–466)

54. (emphasis mine; pg. 21)

55. (www.washingtonpost.com/wp-dyn/content/article/2006/01/24/AR2006012401483.html)

56. (Nathan Batalion, 50 *Harmful Effects of Genetically Modified Foods*)

57. David Williams, Alternatives (For the Health-Conscious Individual; April, 2006 Volume 11, No. 10)

58. (www.newstarget.com/009278.html)

59. (www.msnbc.msn.com/id/12173094)

60. David Williams, *Alternatives (For the Health-Conscious Individual)*; April, 2006 Volume 11, No. 10)

61. (www.timesonline. co.uk/article/0,,3–2128371,00.html)

62. (http://bmj.bmjjournals.com/cgi/content/full/324/7342/886)

63. (www.newstarget.com/009278.html)

64. (Death By Medicine Is American Medicine Working?)

65. (*Journal of the American Medical Association* [JAMA])

66. (*Secrets of the FDA Revealed By Top Insider Doctor*; www.mercola.com/2005/aug/ 13/secrets_of_the_fda_revealed_by_top_insider_doctor.htm)

67. (www.mercola.com/2006/jun/20/ a_novel_way_to_scare_americans_away_from_canadian_drugs.html)

68. (*Secrets of the* FDA *Revealed By Top Insider Doctor*)

69. (www.mercola.com/ 2000/oct/1/FDA_drug_approvals.htm)

70. (www.medicalnewstoday.com/medicalnews.php?newsid=24017)

71. John Robbins, *Diet For A New America* (H.J. Kramer, 1987), 289

72. (www.geocities.com/reflectpool/body.html)

73. www.realage.com)

74. (Carol Krucoff and Mitchell Krucoff, MD, *Healing Moves*, 144)

75. (John Robbins, *A Diet For a New America,* H.J. Kramer, 1987, 110)

Has this book helped and inspired you to make your health a priority? I'd like to hear from you. Contact me at:

inquiries@spirit-of-truth.com.
Web site: www.spirit-of-truth.com

Spirit of Truth Ministries
P.O. Box 755
Hillside, NJ 07205–0755